This book is dedicated with much love to my parents, Rose Marie and Joe Esposito, the greatest parents ever.

TABLE OF CONTENTS

CPSIA information can be obtained
at www.ICGtesting.com
Printed in the USA
BVHW081054091219
566081BV00005B/775/P

9 781633 939769

Eating Right...

For The Health Of It!

By "Dr. Joe" Esposito

Published by Health Plus Publishing
Marietta, Georgia

While a great deal of care has been taken to provide accurate, current, and authoritative information in regard to the subject matter covered in this book, the ideas, suggestions, general principles, conclusions, and any other information presented here are for general education purposes only. This text is sold with the understanding that it is neither designed nor intended to provide the reader with medical or other types of professional health advice. If medical advice or other expert assistance is required, the services of a competent professional should be sought.

Persons who are ill or on medication who wish to change their diet should do so only under the direction of a physician familiar with effects of diet on health.

Printed in the United States of America

Soup-er Recipes ...131

How Sweet It Is! Fruit Meals, Sweets & Snacks 200

INTRODUCTION

When you hear the term vegetarianism, what immediately comes to mind? For many today, it's simply the word to describe the dietary lifestyle they've been leading for any number of years. To another group - vegans - it's a step they passed through some time back on their way to an even purer and healthier way of eating. And finally, for yet one more group - the carnivores among us - though they realize it's something that's probably good for them, it also means sacrifice - giving up their favorite foods. Yikes! Say the word vegan to those who know the meaning but aren't one, and it's an even scarier thought - images of rooting around in the woods for piles of tasteless, boring sticks, roots and assorted shrubbery. Regardless of which of these three groups you happen to fall into, this book is for you. And while "Eating Right... For The Health Of It!" is the first all vegan hypoallergenic cookbook for "kitchen novices," fundamentally, it's about eating well, in many senses of the word, and who among us can't relate to that?

If you're already living the vegetarian or vegan way, you probably swear by the benefits. For those of you who aren't yet, let's start out by defining a few terms.

Different Types of Vegetarians

There are two major types of vegetarians, Lacto-ovo vegetarians and vegans. Lacto and ovo come from the Latin words for milk and egg, respectively, which mean that a lacto-ovo vegetarian will eat eggs and dairy, but no animal flesh. This is a common transition phase that people go through before they become vegan. A vegan (vee-gun) will not eat any animal products, including meat, dairy, eggs, gelatin (which contains animal byproducts), honey, or any other food of animal origin. Many will also avoid any product associated with animals, including leather, certain soaps, cosmetics, cleaning products, etc.

A third level of vegetarians is known as hygenics. This group eats nothing but fruit, vegetables, grains, nuts and seeds. All three have a very wide variety of tasty foods, and all three can easily supply all the nutrients you need to live long and well. And frankly, the closer you are to being a hygenist, the better off you'll be.

For lacto-ovo vegetarians out there considering a transition to veganism, but not sure they want to give up those things that make their style of vegetarianism A-OK, like cheese, ice cream, scrambled eggs, and baked potatoes with butter and sour cream, this cookbook may just show you that indeed, there is life after havarti and loaded spuds. For those just trying to get off the meat wagon, this should open your eyes to the idea that fine dining just doesn't need to include those of the hide, feather, or scale. And for you fellow vegans, "Eating Right... For The Health Of It!" can help you put some pretty dynamic things on your dinner table or nicely supplement your already healthy and environmentally conscience menu. Being a vegan, I have to get a plug in for my dietary choice. Not only will a vegan lifestyle enhance your health like nothing you've ever done before, you'll be eating as well, if not better than you ever have before. So, you're running out of excuses!

Why did I write this book?

I had to write this book. Ever since I was a child I suffered from sinus problems, hives, allergies to just about everything, and was overweight. I think I took every drug known to man in an attempt to "cure" my health problems, yet at best they stayed the same and on bad days I could hardly breathe. I am sure I had what is now known as Attention Deficit Disorder and was in constant trouble in school and at home. My fingers were constantly twitching, my sleep patterns were a mess and my lips and eyes would swell up to the point that it was comical. One day, while in college, I remember waking up and not feeling too bad, but I did not know why. Remembering one of my instructors mentioning that what you eat can have an effect on how you feel, I decided to write down everything I had eaten and done for the previous few days. I realized then that I had, for those days, a very good diet including lots of fruits, vegetables, grains and nuts. I had avoided alcohol, meat, sugar, dairy, coffee, soda and artificial sweeteners. I had lots of rest and a good amount of exercise. So just to be sure, I put back a few of the poisons into my diet and sure enough, I began to feel worse again. This was the beginning of a crusade that would last the rest of my life. I made a commitment to learn and teach others how to prevent disease and treat the cause of illness, not just try to cover up the symptoms. I have been where many of you are, and I understand what you are going through. It is not difficult to change your lifestyle; it is just a different way of living. You have to eat anyway, why not eat good food. This book is designed to teach you how to make simple changes in your life that can make the difference between health and disease, and even life and death. Allow me to teach you to convert to a plant based diet. I promise that once you try it, you will be mad at yourself that you did not do this sooner. It is easy, healthy, a great way to lose weight without "dieting", fun, great for the environment, inexpensive, does not mess up your kitchen as much and will probably add many quality years to your life. If you do not take time to be healthy, you will have to take time to be sick.

For many years, as an adjunct to my chiropractic practice, I have been lecturing professionally on nutrition. If you're into credentials, I have an honors degree in Chiropractic, Diplomate of the American Board of Chiropractic Orthopedics. Diplomate of the American Academy of Pain Management, a BS in clinical nutrition, Diplomate of the College of Clinical Nutrition and Diplomate of the Chiropractic Board of Clinical Nutrition. It's no accident that I chose this arena of study. It is my firm belief that diet, along with a normally functioning nervous system free of interference are the most crucial determinants of long-term health, and in my talks, I discuss how the Standard American Diet (S.A.D.) frankly, does a number on our health. After I finish talking about the subjects so near and dear to our hearts (not to mention stomachs and brains too...), the biggest question is, "So... what do we eat?" The audience wants to know how they can change what they eat without sacrificing taste, convenience, or affordability. They want to know how they can eat fast food or go to a restaurant and still get a nutritious meal. They ask what to put in their pantry and how to stock their refrigerators. They want to know how to eat healthy without going broke or spending half their life in the kitchen. And there's usually someone who wants to know about food allergies and what foods to avoid. This book was written to answer all these questions and more.

Many people genuinely want to change their diet but just aren't sure how. This book will show you how to prepare foods that are delicious, easy to obtain and prepare, environmentally friendly, look good, and most importantly are good for you.

It seemed like an easy task at first: just write down the foods that I eat and put them in a book. What's so hard about that? The problem arose when I realized that many of my favorite foods were from recipes given to me by family and friends, often on a piece of scrap paper or by word of mouth. Some were foods I've eaten since a child and which never followed a recipe - some of this, a little of that, a pinch of the other, etc. Still others were invented over time as my lifestyle changed to a plant-based diet. Each one had to be put into writing in a way that could be easily understood and duplicated.

The book was also inspired by the simple yet often overlooked fact that many people have food "sensitivities"- what we'd call allergies. If you've suffered from a runny nose, digestive problems, fatigue, headaches, rashes, hyperactivity, sleep disturbances, mood swings, weight gain, learning disabilities, mental disorders and even terminal diseases, to name a few, it's often a reaction to what you're eating every day. Did you know that? Now you do. A million light bulbs just went on.

A "Reality" Check

While I know with every fiber of my being that if the world switched to a vegan diet tomorrow, we'd put 90% of the doctors out of business in a few decades, I'm also realistic about the likelihood of that happening anytime soon. And because you're undoubtedly at different places in your dietary evolution, let me make a few disclaimers up front. As you read this, take on those things that make sense for you and that you feel comfortable in adopting. As a vegan, things are pretty cut and dry for me as far as what I will and won't eat, and why. You may not be where I am, and that's fine. So, when I say to definitely avoid this food, that that substance is a poison, or that you should absolutely throw all of this in the trash right now, understand this: Know that I truly believe what I'm saying, and for the sake of your health and that of your family, I want more than anything for you to believe it too, but don't run away because it sounds preachy. Just chuckle to yourself, and say, "Oh, that Dr. Joe." There he goes again with all that scary talk. He's so cute when he gets on his soapbox." Then, take another bite of your hot dog or pizza and keep reading. You'll come around when you're ready.

HOW TO USE THIS BOOK

"Eating Right... For The Health Of It!" is written as a guide to preparing wonderfully tasty and satisfying dishes while avoiding the foods most likely to cause hypersensitivity reactions, the gluten grains: wheat, barley, oats, and rye. Then of course the seven deadly sins of nutrition: alcohol, meat, sugar, dairy, coffee, sodas, and artificial sweeteners. I know, I know, all the good stuff, right? Fear not, we'll get you fed so well, you might just wonder why you never did this sooner. (Because you didn't have a great guidebook like this, remember?)

The pasta recipes in this book call for wheat-free/gluten-free pasta. If you don't have wheat/gluten sensitivity, feel free to use any type of pasta you want. Just keep in mind that I believe that everyone has at least some sensitivity to wheat/gluten. If you don't know whether or not you are sensitive to wheat/gluten, or for that matter any food, start noticing whether you experience excess gas, belching, bloating, sinus problems, fatigue, diarrhea, headaches, dizziness, mood swings, swollen glands, irritability, upset stomach, hives, depression, sneezing, or red eyes (some of the common reactions to foods) after eating wheat. Wheat/gluten can be found in bread, cereal and pasta as well as soy sauce, some soups, gravies, puddings, and lots of other places you might never have thought of. You mean, that could be why I get that reaction, you say? Good possibility. To clear up a few things, let me explain what an allergy is and what sensitivity is. To officially have an allergy, the body must produce certain antibodies in response to consuming a certain food. A diagnosis of allergy is only confirmed after a blood test detects certain antibodies in the blood. Sensitivity is when a person reacts to a certain food, but does not have the antibodies present in their blood. However they may have an increase in white blood cells and/or have a scratch test done in which the skin is scratched and exposed to the suspected problem food. Both blood tests and scratch tests can be misleading, so the easiest, most effective and least expensive way to test if you have a reaction to anything is just avoid the food in question and see how you do.

Options for people with wheat sensitivities are brown and white rice pastas. Then there's corn pasta, potato pasta, and quinoa pasta (pronounced keen-wa.) These pasta options come in a variety of shapes and colors, so try different types until you find your favorite. If you do have a wheat sensitivity and are not sure how you will survive without bread, relax. Tapioca, potato, sorghum, millet and rice breads are available.

Several recipes call for an ingredient called wheat free tamari. Again, this is a hypoallergenic book and this can be replaced with regular tamari sauce. However these contain wheat and often contain hidden MSG. Another alternative can be liquid aminos, which is similar to wheat free tamari and is hypoallergenic.

Some recipes call for a sweetener called rice syrup. You can substitute honey in place of rice syrup, however the recipe is no longer vegan because honey is an animal product. Do not feed honey to infants less than 12 months. Honey can contain bacterial spores that can cause infant botulism. It is a rare disease that affects the nervous system of the infant. Adults and children over the age of 1 are not affected by this condition. (Aw c'mon Joe, ya killin' me here... I warned you, you're talking to a purist. You want honey? Eat honey. Realize of course, that honey is actually.... well...bee vomit. Dig in.)

I also wanted to make the foods with products that you can get at most grocery stores so that preparing a meal can be very convenient and inexpensive, while offering a wide variety of choices. At the same time, you might want to get to know your local natural foods grocery store, complete with their funky clerks, rows of bulk bins, and organic produce. Most large cities have several such establishments. If you've never explored one, it'll be a new experience, and one that will undoubtedly expand your culinary horizons a dimension or two while filling your head with all sorts of ideas for filling your stomach in new and healthy ways. If you're serious about the vegetarian/vegan route, it's a stop you're going to make eventually, and one that will ultimately save you a lot of money.

There are an estimated 120,000 good foods you can eat. This book will help you get the most from a few of them. Use it as a guide, add or subtract spices or ingredients to any or all of these recipes as you see fit. Don't give up on a recipe just because it's not spicy or sweet enough for your liking. Change it to fit your needs and tastes. There's no one right way to make anything. Get creative!

I was going to show how many servings each recipe made in the text; however, there is no standard serving size, and everyone has their own idea of what a serving is. If it was vital to the recipe, the serving size is listed. If not, enjoy your meal and save the rest, if any, for leftovers for the next day. Most recipes will feed 2-4 people, but it depends if this is all you are eating, or you are making more than one food for that particular meal.

When salt is called for, you can substitute lemon juice in the quantity to avoid using salt and still add flavor to the food.

INSTRUCTIONS ON HOW TO EAT

In order to get the most out of what we eat, while steering clear of all sorts of diseases, health problems, and other assorted bad news, we need to watch not only what we eat, but how we eat it. No, we're not talking about new ways to use a knife and fork, but what we might call eating strategies. Such as:

1. Eat only fruit for breakfast. What, no bagel? No egg muffin? I'll just die, you say. Unlikely. Eating fruit will give you all the energy you need while not polluting your body with all that yummy sludge. OK, let me explain. Your body is detoxifying up until about 12 noon and anything but fruit will slow down this process and cause a toxic build up of poisons in your system that can't escape. And thanks to the

high fiber content of fruit, it will also help clean out any waste products built up in your colon.

Anyway, fruit will also supply you with all the nutrients you need to make it through your morning. If you get hungry, eat a handful or two of raw nuts and seeds. Very simple. Bananas are slower to digest than other fruits so they tend to hold off the hunger pangs a little better. If you eat melon, the rule is, "Eat it alone or leave it alone." Melon digestion requires a slightly different level of "stomach juices" than other foods and mixing anything with melon will prevent proper digestion of all the foods. Be sure the fruit you eat is raw and preferably organic. Why organic? Because organic foods are grown without pesticides and in healthy soil which raises their nutritional value. Such a deal. OK, so they're usually a little more expensive, but you're worth it, right? Going organic is especially important for fruits such as apples and peaches where you eat the skin. It's best even with those where you don't eat the skin, like bananas or oranges, though much of the external pesticides are thrown away with the skin. Dried fruits are OK but be sure they don't contain sulfites which are used to make dried fruit look pretty but happen to be toxic. (See the dessert section, most of these can make a great breakfast.) Keep your fruit intake to no more than 3-4 pieces a day.

Trying To Kick The Habit?

If you're a coffee, tea, cola or any other "bad drink" drinker (sorry, just speaking the truth), and you try to give it up all at once - dream on, right? - you may get a headache or general upset feeling. Caffeine withdrawal is not a pleasant experience - for you or those around you. In addition to caffeine having a serious negative on your nervous system, caffeine will block some of the absorption of calcium in your digestive system. Caffeine is often hidden in many foods. Did you know that two aspirin can have as much caffeine as a cup of tea or a glass of cola? If you do want to give it up, put a glass of your favorite caffeinated drink in the refrigerator and every hour that you don't feel good and are just craving some, take one tablespoon of the drink. That should make you feel better. If you feel bad the next hour, repeat the process. If you feel OK the next hour, skip the "fix." Most people report that in 2 to 4 days they can kick the habit. Think of all the money you'll save on that you can now spend on organic produce!

2. Enjoy a wide variety of foods in your diet, but avoid mixing too many different foods in one meal or you'll end up having a hard time properly digesting it all.

3. More and more experts are singing the praises of raw food for one main reason: enzymes. Our bodies desperately need enzymes to process our food efficiently, and raw foods are our only source of this crucial dietary element. So, try to eat at

least one raw food at each meal. Once any food is heated to 110° Fahrenheit or higher, many of the nutrients and enzymes begin to break down. The more we cook our food the less healthy it becomes. A vegetarian/ vegan diet without raw foods is still a long way from healthy. A good variety of raw fruits and veggies spread throughout your day ought to do the trick.

4. Eat as much as you need to keep and maintain a healthy weight and lifestyle, but don't overeat. Too much food dulls and depresses the mind and can cause fatigue, a weakened immune system, and other bad things. Are you reading this after a big meal? Having trouble keeping your eyes open, aren't you?

5. Do not eat meals too close together. Wait until one meal is digested and out of your stomach before piling on another. If the first meal is only partially digested and you dump another pile of food on top of it, the first batch ends up sitting in the stomach too long waiting for the second round to digest so that they both can pass out of the stomach and into the small intestine. And food that sits too long in the stomach gets "over digested" and won't be absorbed very well. Here are a few good rules of thumb.

Before eating again, wait at least:

- 1 hour after eating a fruit-only meal
- 3 hours after eating a starch meal, such as grains or certain vegetables
- 4 hours after eating a protein meal such as beans, nuts, or legumes

Each day add this recipe to whatever you eat, it's good for the digestion and for the soul:

LIFE

1 cup Good Thoughts
1 cup Kind Deeds
1 cup Consideration for Others
2 cups Sacrifice for Others
3 cups Forgiveness
2 cups Well Beaten Faults

Mix these thoroughly and add tears of joy and sorrow and sympathy for others. Fold in 4 cups of love and faith to lighten the other ingredients and raise textures to great heights of positive living. After pouring all this into your daily life, bake well with the warmth of human kindness. Serve with a smile.

What about Allergies and Food Reactions?

Many people suffer from food related allergies. One of the most common allergies is to gluten, which is found in wheat, barley, rye and oats. Symptoms of a gluten allergy include runny nose, gas, diarrhea, and bloating. In children it can also cause ear infections. The best way to test if you have a gluten or other food allergy is to totally avoid the suspected food for five (5) days. On the fifth day, eat a serving or two of those foods, and if you get a reaction, you know to avoid those foods.

Dairy is one thing that all humans are allergic to at some level. Contrary to the ads for dairy digestive aids, lactose-intolerance isn't something that happens to just a few of us. It's estimated that 75%+ of human beings are lactose-intolerant. If that isn't a loud and clear, neon-signed message that we should be avoiding dairy, I don't know what is. Think about it. A looooooooong time ago, someone decided that we were going to consume the milk of another animal. And they built a whole industry around it. And convinced us that the milk made for the young of that species (i.e., calves) was one of the best sources for the nutrients that we humans - a totally different species - needed to build strong bodies. Human beings don't even have the enzyme necessary to digest cow's milk. What a surprise since...hey, we're not cows! Not to mention that the hormone and antibiotic level in processed milk can also lead to allergic reactions. Sort of bizarre, isn't it? So, the moral of the story is, avoid dairy products. And again, I understand that it's probably not going to happen overnight. At least be thinking about phasing it out, an item at a time. And OK, you may never cut it out completely, but the less you have, the better off you'll be. In this book you will find several cows' milk replacements such as almond, coconut, rice, oat, and cashew milk. I think they taste better than cow's milk and are certainly do not cause the negative reactions of cow's milk.

Alcohol is another Hyper-allergenic item. If you're like many people, your sinuses will get nice and stopped up after a few drinks, especially beer and wine. Mild to severe sinus problems are a common side effect of drinking alcohol.

Aspartame and other artificial sweeteners can cause over 92 reactions including headaches, nausea, muscle spasm, blindness, depression, fatigue, memory loss and anxiety to name a few. Do you drink a lot of diet sodas? Do you also get pretty regular headaches? Since aspartame is a vaso-constrictor (tightens the blood vessels), headaches are a pretty predictable reaction. Steer clear of this poison.

And let's not forget MSG (Monosodium Glutamate), the staple seasoning in Chinese food, among other things. Some of the most common reactions from MSG are headaches, difficulty breathing, nausea, vomiting, irregular heartbeat and depression. The tough part about avoiding MSG is that it's often found in many foods but not listed in the ingredients, or even worse, it's referred to as "Natural Flavor." Your own tolerance level to MSG can vary widely from the next guy. While it might take a pile of it to affect him, the smallest amount could trigger a reaction in you. And that reaction could come as soon as immediately after contact all the way up to as much as 48 hours later. Just look how many ways the industry hides this stuff.

These ALWAYS contain MSG:

• Glutamate • Monosodium glutamate • Monopotassium glutamate • Glutamic acid • Calcium caseinate • Sodium caseinate • Gelatin	• Textured protein • Hydrolyzed protein (and any protein that is hydrolyzed) • Yeast extract • Yeast food • Autolyzed yeast • Yeast nutrient

These OFTEN contain MSG

• Malt extract • Malt flavoring • Barley malt • Bouillon • Stock • Broth • Carrageenin • Maltodextrin • Whey protein • Whey protein concentrate • Whey protein isolate • Pectin • Anything protein fortified	• Flavor(s) and Flavoring(s) • Natural flavor(s) and flavoring(s) • Natural pork flavoring • Natural beef flavoring • Natural chicken flavoring • Seasonings (the word "seasonings) • Soy sauce • Soy sauce extract • Soy protein • Soy protein concentrate • Soy protein isolate • Smoke flavoring

Hidden MSG is not limited to foods. MSG sensitive people have reported reactions to soaps, shampoos, hair conditioners, and cosmetics that contain MSG. The most common obvious hiding places are in ingredients called "hydrolyzed protein" and "amino acids", although not all amino acids contain MSG.

Drinks, candy and chewing gum are also potential sources of MSG. Also aspartic acid, found in aspartame, has been reported to cause MSG type reactions in MSG sensitive people. Aspartame is also found in some medications so it is a good idea to check with your pharmacist.

Binders and fillers for medication, nutrients and supplements, both prescription and non-prescription, including some food formulas and some fluids administered intravenously in hospitals, may contain MSG.

Even good food can often cause adverse reactions in certain people. Strawberries, pineapples, tomatoes, grapefruits, and oranges are common culprits in causing hives, skin rash, and more often, outbreaks on the tongue and lips.

As a side note, sometimes suspected food allergies or sensitivities can be just reactions to fabric softeners, deodorant soaps or detergents touching the skin and producing rashes or other symptoms. If you have a reaction to a certain food or product, simply avoid it. This book is written to show you how you can eat well, live a normal life, and avoid most common allergic reactions.

A DIET TO GROW ON

As plant-based diets become more popular, the public is rapidly becoming aware of the dangers of eating animal products such a meat, dairy and eggs and their by-products.

There are plenty of terrifying tales about what goes into the raising and processing of livestock and poultry. I won't ruin your appetite now, since that would sort of defeat my purpose here, but suffice it to say that steroids, chemicals, hormones, antibiotics and tranquilizers, commonly used in raising beef and poultry, have found their way onto dinner plates across the country. Many people consider the way animals are raised and slaughtered inhumane. It is not so important as to why you stop eating flesh, it is important that you do.

The emergence and growth of products such as free range chicken and chemical-free beef reflects both Americans' growing awareness of these new dangers as well as a demand for healthy substitutes. However even those "healthy" substitutes do not digest well and can cause a number of serious and deadly health problems.

People everywhere are choosing to fill their dinner plates with vegetarian foods instead of the traditional elements of the food chain. Yet some health practitioners still feel that this healthy lifestyle is unsafe or unwise for children. Yet, it would seem logical that children, whose immune systems are generally not as strong as adults, would benefit from a non-animal product containing diet.

According to the American Dietetic Association, "Infants, children, and adolescents who consume well balanced vegetarian diets can generally meet all their nutritional requirements for growth." The ADA endorses a vegetarian diet, concluding that the nutrients found in animal products can also be found in a plant based diet. Imagine that.

And to stay on my soapbox for a little bit longer, when it comes to nutrition in this country, we seem to have lost our common sense and our better judgment. In fact, all we've gained are unhealthy eating habits and a lot of weight!

I want to take a few minutes here and talk about the right diet for children, from newborns all the way through teenagers. As if you didn't have enough to do just dealing with teenagers, now you have to mess with their diets too? Or perhaps you do not have kids. No problem. Just skip this section and move on to bigger, better, and more delicious topics. We'll catch up with you shortly.

FEEDING YOUR CHILD FROM BIRTH TO THE TEEN YEARS

The Right Diet For New Mother and Baby

Many common health problems among babies including digestive disorders, and respiratory illnesses are actually reactions to certain foods, especially animal based foods.

There's little debate that the ideal food for infants is mother's milk, which contains all the necessary nutrients including water, carbohydrates, fats, protein, vitamins, and minerals to nourish the infant up to the first two years. Mother's milk helps to build the child's immune system, assists in normal cell growth and mental maturation, and helps build a bond between mother and child. Yet, amazingly, the formula industry has somehow convinced new mothers (the formula kits sitting invitingly by their hospital bedsides are as subtle as a 2 x 4) that their product is just as good if not better than the wondrous creation that is mother's milk, despite the fact that we're still discovering how miraculous mother's milk really is. Oh well.

The most important time to breast feed is immediately after birth. The first milk, called colostrum, is slightly yellow. It is a super concentrated form of nutrients designed to 1) help the baby nutritionally, 2) act as a laxative to clean out the newborn's gastrointestinal tract, and 3) provide healthy bacteria (flora) and antibiotics to prepare the baby for digestion of solid foods. The colostrum will slowly change to regular breast milk by the third week.

During breast feeding the mothers diet must be healthy. It is important that the mother takes care of herself while she's feeding the baby. Studies have shown that vegetarian moms have a lower level of pesticides in their milk than women who eat the standard American diet. There is no substitute for the greatest nutritional gift of all - breast feeding.

However, if a mother is unable to breast feed, breast milk may be purchased from other nursing mothers who make their extra milk available to infants who may not get breast milk any other way. (Information on obtaining breast milk may be obtained by calling the local La Leche League.)

Or, if a baby needs formula, use organic formula only. Other types may lead to digestive problems and allergies. Children not breast fed seem to have more allergic reactions to food and environmental conditions as adults than those children who are breast-fed. Gee, what a surprise.

OK, so when is an infant ready to start adding solid food to their diet? One guidepost is when the baby has doubled his or her birth weight and the child needs to be fed more than 8 – 10 times per day. It is a good idea to continue to breast feed as usual while you add solid foods. This process can begin as early as 7 months, as late as 12 months and can continue for up to 2 years.

When you decide to introduce solid foods, breast-feeding can now be supplemented with cereals, mashed fruits and/or vegetables. It is important to introduce solid foods one at a time to reduce the risk of allergic reactions. It is widely accepted that brown rice cereal be the first solid food which is introduced to the infant. It is not recommended that you use wheat, barley, corn, oats, or rye cereals. These can cause allergic reactions such as gas, diarrhea, pimples, hyperactivity, mood swings, ticklishness, and repetitive rhythmical motions in your infant. If your child has any of these symptoms at any age, a food allergy just might be the reason.

To make the cereal, prepare 1/3 cup of a thin consistency of cereal and milk (rice or breast milk). Feed this to your child once a day. Increase gradually to 1/2 cup. As the baby requires more food, go to 2 meals a day consisting of 1/4 to 1/2 cup per meal.

Soft fruit may also be used as a baby's first solid food. Ripe bananas, avocado, apples, peaches, or pears may be mashed or pureed, ideally in a food processor. Be careful with strawberries or kiwi, as these can often cause reactions such as diaper rash or tongue lesions. So, keep an eye out, and if these reactions occur, simply avoid that food.

There is a debate over whether to introduce cereals or fruit as the first food. Either one seems fine. However, only introduce one food at a time every 2 to 3 weeks.

Vegetables may also be introduced beginning at 7 to 10 months, depending on your child. Carrots, peas, sweet potatoes, and green beans should be cooked and mashed well. Cooked lentils and split peas are good, but may cause gas. One problem with cooked food is that once the food is heated above 110° many of the nutrients are destroyed, whereas fruits served in their raw, natural state have all their nutrients.

There is no reason to season these foods when introducing them to your child. You might not like the taste (and if you did, you might not want to tell too many people...), but actually babies are quite happy with non-seasoned foods. Since many seasonings such as sugar, salt and spices can have negative effects on your baby's health; go easy - if at all.

Vegetables may be used in addition to, but not in place of, fruit. Tofu, another great choice, is hypoallergenic and a great source of iron, calcium, and protein. Choose tofu processed with calcium sulfate, as it's easier to digest.

Do not mix fruits and vegetables in the same meal. They do not digest well together and can prevent proper absorption of both foods. By mixing foods, you also make it more difficult to determine which foods your child may not like or to what foods he or she may be allergic.

While some experts recommend breads, crackers or dried cereals as early as 6 months, I'd suggest waiting until at least the 12 month mark. When you introduce breads, crackers and dried cereals, avoid wheat, oats, rye, barley and corn. Many children have very subtle allergies to these foods. Better choices include rice, tapioca, potato, sorghum or millet breads, crackers or cereals.

Nut butters such as almond and cashew may be introduced as early as 12 months. Add coconut, rice or breast milk to thin the butters and make them more digestible. Be sure not to give too large a serving, as the baby can choke on nut butters. Caution: Avoid peanut butter since many children have peanut allergies. Note: Other foods to be careful with are whole grapes, popcorn, whole nuts, and small, hard pieces of fruit and vegetables because they can get lodged in the throat.

Your happy, healthy one year old should be breast feeding and eating the following daily:

- 4 servings of cereals/breads (1 serving = 1/4 slice of gluten free bread or

  2-4 tablespoon of cereal)
- 4 servings of fruit and vegetables (1 serving = 1-6 tablespoon of fruit and/or vegetables)
- 2 servings of legumes and nut butters (1 serving = 1/4 oz.)

As your child becomes a toddler and pre-teen, the same "adult" rules apply: lots of fruits, vegetables, grains, and nuts. As long as your child is getting enough calories and volume to support good energy levels and normal growth, he or she should be getting an adequate supply of all the necessary nutrients for optimum growth and function.

GETTING ENOUGH B12?

One important issue is the question of vitamin B12 and how much supplementation, if any, is needed in a totally plant-based diet. While some studies show adequate B12 in fruits, especially organic fruits, and that no supplementation is needed, be on the safe side and make sure you have a reliable source of B12 in your diet. What is the best source? Inexpensive and great-tasting nutritional yeast fortified with B12 (Read the ingredients on the label to be sure you have good quality yeast).

Unlike other kinds of yeast that may cause infections and other health problems, you'll have no problems with nutritional yeast. Not only is it a great source for the entire B complex, it's loaded with many other vitamins, minerals, and amino acids – the building blocks of all proteins. It comes in a flaky, powdery form and is great sprinkled on salad, popcorn, pasta and rice dishes, pizza and soups. Be sure to add it after the food is cooked because cooking with it can destroy much of its nutritional value. With an almost cheese-like flavor, it's not only good for you, but can be used as a seasoning. Add about 1 tablespoon of nutritional yeast to your child's and your own food 2 to 3 times per week for all the B12 you need. Other good sources of B12 are fortified non-dairy milk or a B12 supplement.

Concerned about protein and calcium? The fact is, the average person of any age rarely has a problem getting enough protein. As long as they are eating enough good foods to give them sufficient calories to maintain their growth and energy level, protein shouldn't be a problem. And as a rule, we're getting way far too much animal protein in our diets. While it's my contention (and the facts bear it out) that we need zero animal protein to be healthy, do what works for you and just be cognizant of the reality.

As far as calcium goes, be sure you eat 3 or more servings of foods per day that supply calcium and you'll be just fine. These include but are not limited to tofu, tahini (sesame butter), green, leafy vegetables such dark green lettuces, broccoli, collard greens, mustard greens, most nuts and kale. If you are not eating the high acid foods such as meats, dairy products (supposedly high sources of calcium, right?) and sodas you will require less calcium than the average person. More acid in your diet means more calcium is being excreted from your body, which ups your calcium requirements.

PRE-TEEN AND TEENAGE YEARS

I know, just getting pre-teens and teenagers to eat anything can be a challenge, much less trying to get them to cut back or eliminate all the other junk they seem so enamored with such as the four basic teen food groups: pizza, potato chips, pastries and slurpees. Talk about sending shivers up your spine... Short of a seat with arm straps, a crowbar and a funnel, just do the best you can. As always, and of course, ideally, alcohol, meat, sugar, dairy, coffee, soda and artificial sweeteners should be avoided. The volume of food will need to increase to meet the rapid growth they are experiencing. Many teens, especially girls, lean toward a low fat diet due to weight concerns (and isn't that the understatement of the century...). This can have dangerous consequences. The body requires fat for proper production of hormones. Teaching teens that there are good fats and bad fats can help. Teach them to avoid hydrogenated oils, milk, cheese and animal products and replace them with better choices such as vegetable oil, cheese-free gluten free pizza, non-dairy milk, "burgers" made with no meat, gluten free bread and burger toppings without the meat, salads, stir fried vegetables or tofu at a Chinese restaurant or gluten free pasta with a marinara sauce instead of a meat sauce. This will give the teen the freedom to be a kid, yet not poison themselves every time they go out with their friends. By starting early with good eating habits, you'll make healthier eating part of their lifestyle.

Acknowledge that not all of their friends - very few in fact -, will think like them when it comes to food, and that by eating healthy, they'll be really "different"! (We all know how important that is to teenagers...) Tell them that the best way to educate their peers is by example, and of course, you educate them by example. Have lots of quality snacks around the house such as fruits, nuts, seeds, dried fruit (without sulfites), nut butters, air popped pop corn, and rice cakes. These will give them plenty of food and allow for a normal growth pattern without too much concern about being overweight. Make sure you tell them that eating healthy can even control or eliminate acne. Whatever it takes. Sometimes, you gotta pull out the big guns here. My job is giving you the right advice, the healthy advice. Practical? Realistic? Up to you. The ball's in your court.

In teenagers, like in children, watch for signs of allergies. Runny nose, mood swings, nervousness, hyperactivity, itching, swelling, rashes, gas, and bad breath can all be signs of food allergies. The easiest way to find out what a person is allergic to is to totally eliminate one food at a time from the diet for at least 5 days. On the fifth day, reintroduce the food in question. If the adverse reaction occurs, you can safely assume you're sensitive to that food and you need to avoid it. If you suspect that a food allergy exists, as we discussed earlier, start with some very common allergens such as wheat, oats, barley, corn, strawberries, grapefruit and dairy (which of course, you've already eliminated, right? Just checkin'). And do not forget that some people have reactions to certain clothes and regular soaps, perfumes, unclean air, dust and air fresheners. OK, we're going to cut back on our gloom and doom and talk about what is good and getting your kitchen ready for the new you.

LOTS OF PASTABILITIES

As you'll soon find out, many recipes in this and other books include pasta, certainly a favorite staple of the American diet. Wide variety, versatile, easy to prepare, and good for you, pasta is a winner. Of course, in this cookbook, you'll find recipes for only wheat free/gluten free pasta. And luckily for you, you've got lots of choices. A few tips for wheat free pasta: It's important to cook wheat free pasta in a little more water than regular pasta or it can get mushy. A good rule to follow is 6 quarts of water to 1 pound of pasta. As far as sauce goes, a good rule is 3 cups of sauce per pound of pasta. Feast your eyes:

Brown rice pasta - popular and very tasty. Close to wheat pasta, but not as sticky. Generally tolerated by anyone so if you have a wheat sensitivity, serve this to your friends and you'll enjoy the meal as well.

Corn pasta has a subtle corn flavor which makes it a great choice for vegetable and bean dishes. And while many people have corn allergies, it's not nearly as common as wheat allergies.

Quinoa-corn pasta - a mixture of quinoa and corn that increases the protein content of corn pasta. Quinoa has a slightly nutty flavor. Those with corn allergies may not do well with this one. While you should be able to find some of these pastas in your local grocery store, your health food store will certainly have a wider and more readily available variety

KITCHEN HINTS

- Keep your pantry well stocked.
- Keep a running shopping list so when you are almost out of an item, you know to buy more.
- Be sure to have a clean space to prepare your meals. It's not only more sanitary, it makes it easier as well.
- Keep spices in the cooking area for easy access but away from the heat.
- Keep utensils handy and your knives sharp. Since steak knives don't cut very well, it's a good idea to invest in sharp, high quality stainless steel kitchen knives.
- Have a large cutting board.
- If a recipe calls for boiling water start boiling it before beginning the rest of the preparation.
- Make more than you'll eat at one meal, and then freeze the leftover meals for quick meals later.
- Cook for a friend. Life is more fun when you share.
- Set a timer if you get easily side-tracked, to remind yourself of what to do when.

- The more often you prepare food, the easier it gets, so practice, practice, practice!

Stocking and Unstocking Your Pantry

The first rule of eating right is "Get the Junk Out of the House." If lousy, unhealthy food is in the house, you'll eat it. Stock only good healthy food that will nourish your body. Don't say, "As soon as I eat the stuff I have, I'll get new healthy stuff." Get rid of it right now. Stop reading and... OK, you promise you'll do it later? Don't be sneaking a doughnut when I'm looking the other way... Fill up your pantry with good stuff like I have listed below. For some of you, the list will be old news, but a lot of the items will be new to many of you. But, hey, that's what this adventure is all about, right? Just try them. If you don't like 'em, don't eat them. That's what's so great about this country. You never have to do anything you don't want to, in most cases.

Grains

This category includes different types of rice such as Brown, Basmati, and Long Grain. Avoid the white rice. It's processed and void of many of its natural nutrients. Sorghum, quinoa, millet, corn grits and wild rice are good staples to start with once you get a little adventurous. I also recommend that you try buckwheat, teff, and nut flours. As for storage of the grains, keep them in a well-sealed glass or plastic container. Add a bay leaf to the jars in the pantry to help keep the bugs away. If your pantry is hot, keep your grains in the refrigerator. Label all containers.

When you're learning a bunch of new foods, the last thing you need is to have to figure out whether that's the quinoa or the millet in that jar. In addition to labeling them, take a minute and write out basic directions for their preparation and tape it to the side of the container or on the inside of the lid. When brown rice takes 50 minutes to prepare and couscous takes five, it's a good idea not to get the two confused. On to the beans...

Beans and Legumes

Chick Peas, Pinto Beans, Great Northern Beans, Cannellini Beans, Green and Yellow Split Peas, Red and Brown Lentils, and Black Beans are all excellent choices to add to your diet, providing high levels of protein, fiber, and they give you the "full" feeling that you were accustomed to when you were a meat eater. Place beans and legumes in sealed containers, preferably glass or plastic, label them, and store in a cool dry place.

Pasta

Keep on hand rice pasta, quinoa pasta and corn pasta, all of which come in a variety of shapes and colors and have wonderfully interesting textures and flavors. Remember, this book is written with a hypoallergenic theme. Processed white flours which are used to make most conventional stiff, plastic wrapped pastas, are not digested well, and can cause runny nose, mucus in the body, gas, and fatigue - while draining your body of vital nutrients. Besides, white flour pasta is borrrrrrring. Even if you do not have an adverse reaction to wheat, these other pastas are tastier and much more fun. Store pasta in a cool dry place in well-sealed containers.

Sea Veggies

Dulse and Nori - yes, they're seaweed - are great seasonings for salad, soups and dressings, as well as popcorn, potatoes, stir fries and beans. Not used to eating seaweed? Think again. Within kelp - the "monster" seaweed that blankets large sections of the ocean floor - is a sticky gum-like substance called algin that ends up in hundreds of foods as a thickener, along with many other products. Algin keeps ice cream "creamy"and improves the smoothness and texture of cake frosting. Thanks to algin in salad dressing, the oil and vinegar stay together a lot longer. Algin puts the "glaze" in glazed doughnuts, makes milkshakes velvety, whipped cream silky and pancake syrup thick. Slow-moving ketchup? Blame it on the algin! Of course, you won't be eating many of those foods anymore, will you?

If you swim in the ocean and eat animals from the ocean, what's the big deal about seaweed? These sea vegetables are slightly salty in flavor and are loaded with nutrients including vitamin B12. These are seasonings that may not be part of your menu now, but once you try them you will most likely make them part of your usual flavor enhancers.

Nuts and Seeds

Almonds, cashews, pecans, filberts, walnuts, pine nuts, sunflower seeds, sesame seeds and pumpkin seeds are just some of the nutritious selections you have to choose from. Be sure to choose nuts that are raw, since when they're roasted, they loose valuable nutrients. Nuts and seeds, once shelled, will last about 4-6 months if refrigerated, up to one year if frozen.

Nut and Seed Butters

Almond, peanut, cashew, sesame (also called Tahini) and sunflower make excellent butters. These can be bought commercially or made at home in your blender or food processor. Nut and seed butters require refrigeration after opening and will last up to four months.

Dried Fruits

Raisins, figs, apples, mango, papaya, dates, banana, prunes, apricots pears, peaches persimmon, pineapple, coconut and tomatoes are all great to eat when dried. Be on the lookout for and avoid those containing sulfites or added sugar. Store dried fruits in airtight glass or plastic containers, in a cool, dry place, and they'll keep up to six months. If you prefer, soak fruits in distilled warm water for an hour before eating. This is a nice alternative but certainly isn't necessary. If you want to get real ambitious and have a lot of fun in the process, you can pick up a food dehydrator. Make your own dried fruit, using organic fruit and then you'll know what you're eating.

Dried Spices and Herbs

Basil, bay leaves, red pepper, black pepper, cayenne pepper, poultry seasoning, cilantro, garlic, ginger, oregano, turmeric, rosemary, sage, tarragon, thyme, savory, dill weed, chili powder, chives, cinnamon, nutmeg, paprika. Store in a cool, dry, convenient place, in sealed glass or plastic containers.

Fats and Oils

Poor fat. What a bad rap it's gotten in the last few years. Sure, on average we Americans consume too much of it, but when we get so obsessed with a low fat or no fat diet, things can get out of hand and some people have reduced their fat intake to unhealthy levels. Bottom line, we need fats in our diets. There have been many fat-free diets and products made available to the public, and most are, at best, not very healthy and at worst, downright dangerous. And by the way, fat-free doesn't mean calorie free. I have to chuckle - sadly - when I hear stories about people who just plow through a whole box of fat-free cookies in one sitting and when questioned, reply, "But, they're fat-free!" You've never done that, have you? I don't want to know.

We need fat to produce the walls around our cells, give us energy stores, help insulate the body, make hormones, and a host of other functions. There's good fat and bad fat. The bad fats are saturated or hydrogenated fats. If a product says hydrogenated or partially hydrogenated oil, avoid it. These dangerous fats will not only cause hardening of the arteries, but they'll hijack the good fats in your body and use them to transport and metabolize them. This could lead to not having enough good fats.

Use organic, unrefined oils purchased in small amounts to avoid spoilage. Keep in a dark place as sunlight can destroy many nutrients in oils. You can keep oil in the refrigerator and while it may become thick and cloudy, this is fine and won't affect its use. The best oils for salads are Olive, Coconut and Flax. The best oil for very light sautéing, sauces and salads is olive oil. Keep olive oil and coconut oil on hand. When you get brave, try other oils such as sesame, avocado, almond, grape seed, or sunflower.

Beverages

Naturally caffeine-free herbal teas, coconut milk, rice milk, almond milk, 100% fruit juice (in small quantities), seltzer (not to be confused with club soda which has quite a bit of unhealthy salt in it), and good old plain distilled or filtered water. Store teas in a cool dry place. Once juices and milks are open they generally only last a week or two. If a drink or food smells or tastes bad, throw it away. Another one of the benefits of pre packaged rice and other non-dairy milks is that they'll last longer in the refrigerator than cow's milk will. And until you open them, you can store them in your pantry, unrefrigerated, which is great if you find a killer deal and want to buy a whole case of the stuff. You'll get used to the new types of milk and the old cow's milk will not even taste good before long. An even healthier choice is to make your own milks. There are several recipes in this book to show you how. Try different types of milks, use the ones you like and do not use the others. All the milks in this book are good choices.

Experiment with a juicer and make your own juice or just purchase them commercially.

Salty Seasonings

Sea salt, wheat free Tamari (similar flavor to soy sauce), miso, Bragg's Liquid Aminos, olives. Storage: Refrigerate miso, others can be kept at room temperature.

Other Seasonings and Such

Rice Vinegar, balsamic vinegar, apple cider, salsa, vegan mayonnaise (contains no eggs or hydrogenated oil), ketchup that is made without sugar, capers, hot sauce, mustard, lemon juice, lime juice, vanilla. Store vinegar at room temperature, the others require refrigeration.

What about Pots and Pans & other Equipment?

Ceramic, cast iron and stainless steel are the best. If you're going to use non-stick cookware, be sure to use the best quality available. Cheap non-stick and coated pans can easily scratch and bits of this toxic coating can end up in your food. Aluminum and copper cookware can also get into your food causing toxic symptoms.

A food processor is a big help with most things. Just remember you get what you pay for. A quality machine will process your food, release nutrients, and make food preparation easier for many years. Have a variety of plastic and glass containers available for storage or supplies and leftovers. Spatulas, mixing bowls and a colander are a must for any well equipped kitchen. It is imperative to have good sharp knives and a large cutting board.

What to do if a recipe just doesn't taste right

- Try adding a little more of each seasoning, one at a time. You can always add more, but removing it is a bit trickier.
- If it is too salty, add more of the other ingredients, such as oil, grains, or liquid.
- If it's too sweet, try adding a little lemon juice, salt or oil.
- If the meal gets burned, don't stir it. Just use the unburned part and toss the rest. Waste not, want not.
- Remember: a recipe is nothing more than a guideline. Get brave, experiment with new things, change ingredients or add things you like. Who knows, maybe you'll write your own cookbook before long.

Dining "a la car"

Note: some of these choices may not be ideal, such as white rice or hydrogenated oil contained in the food, but this is "nutrition for the real world." If you have Celiac disease or gluten intolerance, I recommend carrying a dining card with you that you can show your server to more easily explain your dietary needs. Here is an example of one that you can copy and carry with you:

I have an illness called Celiac Disease and have to follow a strict Gluten Free Diet. I will become very ill if I eat even a crumb of gluten, so please read the following carefully.

Gluten is found in many food items, but most commonly in flours and grains of wheat (durum, semolina, kamut, spelt), rye, barley and some oats.

Foods that may contain gluten include soy sauce, blue cheese, breading, imitation bacon, marinades, processed meats, soup bases, thickeners, broth, croutons, gravies, imitation seafood, pastas, stuffings, salad preservatives etc.

Foods that are safe include unseasoned and marinated meats, fruit, veggies, eggs, cheese, milk, rice, corn, potato, bean, sorghum, quinoa, millet, buckwheat, arrowroot, amaranth, teff and nut flours.

In addition to being aware of the above ingredients, please take care to make sure my food is not contaminated by other food containing gluten by doing the following:

- Prepare my food in a **clean area** on a clean surface.
- Wash your hands and **wear clean gloves** while preparing my food.
- Use only **clean utensils** including strainers, tongs, knifes, spoons.
- Use only **clean water and oil** in clean dishes when preparing my food – do not use water that has cooked wheat pasta and do not use oil that has had wheat food fried in it such as breaded chicken fingers.
- Do not cut my food on a cutting board that has had bread on it.
- Do not wash my fruit or drain my pasta in a strainer that has been used to drain pasta.

- If grilling food, thoroughly **clean the grill** with a metal brush before placing my food on the grill. Marinades often contain gluten.
- If you accidentally add croutons to my salad, please do not just remove them from the salad. I can still get sick from the contamination of the salad by the croutons. Please prepare me a new salad.
- Only use new **clean tubs of condiments** such as butter, mayo, mustard and ice cream. Previously used tubs may have been contaminated by a utensil that had gluten on it – such as a butter knife or ice cream scooper that was used for a flavor containing a gluten ingredient.
- Do not season my food unless we have discussed the seasonings – use only salt and pepper and no garnish on my plate unless it is fresh and has no sauce.
- Most importantly, when in doubt go without!! If you are unsure about something, please do not serve it to me without asking.

Mexican

Make sure the beans aren't made with lard (a pretty common practice), just ask the waiter.

Bean tacos
Bean tamales
Bean tostados
Potato enchiladas
Bean enchiladas
Beans, salsa and guacamole with chips (chips made
with non genetically modified (GMO) corn)

Chinese

Remember to ask for no MSG, soy sauce, and chicken or beef broth. Most dishes can be made vegetarian, and gluten free, so ask for it if you want it. Carry your own wheat free tamari, many restaurants will cook your meal with it if you ask them.

Stir-fried vegetables
Vegetable fried rice (with wheat free tamari)
Broccoli and peas
Any vegetable tofu meal
Rice noodles
Steamed vegetables

Thai

Like Chinese, be sure there is no MSG, fish sauce (it can contain MSG), soy sauce, chicken or beef broth.
And since most dishes can be made vegetarian and gluten free, just ask.

Curry vegetables
Curry tofu
Mixed vegetables
Vegetable fried rice
Pad Thai

Italian

Strangely enough, some restaurants will use a beef or chicken broth base in their "meatless" sauces, so be sure to ask about it. Some restaurants carry wheat free/gluten free pasta or will let you bring your own, just ask.

Wheat Free/Gluten Free Pasta with tomato sauce
Wheat Free/Gluten Free Pasta with pesto sauce (no cheese)

Salad
Broccoli rabe (rappini)
Pizza on gluten free crust (some restaurants carry these or will let you bring your own) with no cheese (top it with sauce, tomatoes, mushrooms, peppers, onions, etc.)

Japanese

Again, bring your own wheat free tamari.

Salad
Avocado sushi
Mushroom sushi
Any other vegetable sushi
Yakatori (grilled vegetables or tofu on a stick)
Teppen vegetable dinner (this is that "chop-chop, sizzle sizzle" style of dining where they cook the food in front of you.)

American

Salads/Salad bar
Baked potatoes plain or topped with things such as salsa, salad dressing, guacamole, tomato sauce, etc.
Almond butter, or cashew butter and all fruit jelly sandwich on wheat free/gluten free bread
Corn on the cob
Fresh fruit

Other options include; Indian, Pakistan, or Korean food. Just be sure they are made wheat free/gluten free, and with no animal products.

Hint: If you're really stumped, look at the side orders and pick a few of the more enticing choices from that list and make a meal of them.

Refrigeration, ripening, and freshness tips

- Keep dried goods such as flours, grains, dried fruits and spices in jars to avoid bugs and to help keep them organized.
- Wrap leafy vegetables in a paper towel, then place in a plastic bag to keep them moist and help them last longer.
- Always buy organic whenever possible. Organic means the product was grown in a healthy soil free of pesticides. The produce is usually much tastier, has up to 70% more nutrients than non organic produce and is better for the environment. The down side is it may cost a little more and may not be as pretty as non-organic produce. And when people say they can't afford organic, my response is, "You can't afford not to buy organic." (What else would I say?) The "buy organic" idea is especially true for fruits that you eat the skin, such as apples or peaches, and root vegetables such as potatoes, carrots, and turnips because if you weren't able to wash all the dirt off the food before you eat it, it wouldn't be nearly as damaging as if you ate non-organic food. It is best to eat the skins of fruits or vegetables that have edible skins because many important nutrients are found in and just below the skin. I would not recommend eating the skin of a non organic root vegetable. Better yet, grow your own garden. It is less expensive and fresh is best.
- Make sure you're eating ripe fruit, since the nutritional value of ripe fruit is much higher than when the fruit is not fully ripened. Fruit is usually ripe when you gently push on it and it feels slightly soft, similar to pushing on the tip of your nose.

Don't refrigerate unripe fruit. Once it's been refrigerated, it inhibits the ripening process.

- To ripen fruit like bananas, avocados, and tomatoes better and faster, place them in a brown paper bag. Just be sure to check them daily, because the process goes fast once it starts. We don't want to be too successful and end up throwing it out. Bananas are ripe when they have a few brown speckles on them. Once they get this ripe, eat up, since they'll only last a few days.
- Vegetables and fruits last longer if they are not washed until just before they are to be used.
- When using only a portion of an onion, save the root end, it will last longer.
- When just a little lemon juice is needed, stick it with a fork and squeeze instead of cutting the whole lemon, it will last longer.
- Place a raw potato, a slice of bread or an open box of baking soda in the refrigerator. These will absorb odors.
- Purchase pre-chopped garlic because it's just a whole lot easier. You can find it in glass jars in the produce section of your grocery store.

Note: Some folks say just fruit for breakfast leaves them hungry. If you are hungry after an hour or two eat 1-2 handfuls of nuts or seeds! Wait at least an hour or two so the first fruit can get out of your stomach. Don't pile one meal on top of another. Non fruit meals take 4 to 6 hours to get out of your stomach.

7 Breakfasts

1. Fruit Shake
   1 banana
   1 cup fruit juice (apple, peach, orange, etc...)
   1 apple
   10 grapes

Mix in blender. (Get crazy, try frozen fruits or freeze the banana after peeling and cutting in thirds. See the famous breakfast shake recipe for more shake ideas.)

2. Fruit Salad
   3 strawberries
   1 orange
   1 apple

Cut in pieces and mix.

3. Melon Bowl
   1/2 cantaloupe cubed
   1/2 honeydew cubed

Mix together and enjoy! (With melons it is best to eat them alone or leave them alone. They digest differently than other fruits and this is why this concept is important.)

4. Tropical Treat
   1/2 small papaya peeled and cubed
   1 cup pineapple cubed
   1/2 cup shredded coconut

Mix and eat.

5. Fruit Balls

    1/2 cup raisins
    1/2 cup dates, mashed
    1 ripe banana
    1 apple or pear diced

Mash banana. Add rest of fruit. Roll in balls place on cookie sheet cover with wax paper and refrigerate until hard. Enjoy!

6. Banana Ice Cream

See page 217 for recipe.

7. Fruit Pie

See page 208-210 for recipes.

7 Lunches

1. Spinach pesto over brown rice or pasta
   Arugula salad with cucumbers dressing
   Seltzer
2. Oriental Patties
   Spinach Salad with Tahini-miso dressing
3. Vegetarian Chile
   Mixed field greens with peach salad dressing
4. Creamy carrot Soup
   Beet salad with scallions
5. Potato Pancakes with an apple sauce or vegan sour cream
   Cucumber salad
6. Gazpacho Soup
   Eggless egg salad
7. Black Bean Salad
   Roasted potatoes Cajun style

7 Dinners

1. Eggplant salad
   Sun dried tomatoes poured over brown rice

2. Curried lentils and spinach
   Green Goddess dressing over sliced cucumbers

3. Asparagus mushrooms risotto
   Dr. Joe's Signature salad

4. Mom Esposito's Macaroni and Beans
   Tomato basil salad

5. Black bean salad
   Carrot soup with cilantro

6. Pesto Potatoes Wedges
   Lettuce with Italian dressing

7. Tomato Basil sauce over pasta or brown rice
   Spinach with lemon tarragon dressing

WATER OR SELTZER TO DRINK

Some Helpful Cooking Tips...

Grain Cooking Times

Grain (dry cups)	Water (cups)	Cooking Time	Yield
Amaranth	1½ – 2½	20-25 minutes	2
Basmati (brown)	2	45 minutes	3
Basmati (white)	1¾	15-20 minutes	2½
Brown Rice	2	1 hour	3
Buckwheat (kasha)	2	15 minutes	2½
Coarse Cornmeal (polenta)	4	25 minutes	3
Millet	2	30 minutes	4
Teff	4	15-20 minutes	2
Wild Rice	2½	50-60 minutes	4
Quinoa	2	15 minutes	3

Table of Equivalents

1 teaspoon = ⅓ tablespoon = 5 milliliters

1 ½ teaspoons = ½ tablespoon

3 teaspoons = 1 tablespoon = 15 milliliters

4 tablespoons = ¼ cup = 59 milliliters

5 ⅓ tablespoons = ⅓ cup = 79 milliliters

8 tablespoons = ½ cup = 118.4 milliliters

16 tablespoons = 1 cup

1 cup = 8 fluid ounces = .2366 liters (approx. ¼ liter)

2 cups = 1 pint = .4372 liters (approx. ½ liter)

4 cups = 2 pints = 1 quart = .9463 liters (approx. 1 liter)

4 quarts = 1 gallon

1 ounce = approx. 28 grams

3 ½ ounces = 100 grams

16 ounces = 1 pound

1 pound = 454 grams

2.2 pounds = 1 kilogram

OK, LET'S GET COOKIN'!

Entertaining Entrées

PASTA IN A PINK SAUCE

12-16 oz. wheat free/gluten free pasta

8 sun-dried tomatoes in oil

Handful of fresh parsley (1/2 cup)

1/2 cup water

1 clove garlic, peeled

6 fresh basil leaves (or 1 tsp. dried)

1/2 pound firm tofu

3 Tbsp. olive oil

Pine nuts and parsley, for garnish

Prepare pasta as directed on the box. Place tomatoes, parsley, water, garlic, basil, and tofu in food processor. Blend 30 seconds, then add olive oil in a slow steady stream while still blending. Pour into a medium saucepan and cook gently over low heat, about 10 minutes. Add pasta to boiling water and cook uncovered until tender, about 10 minutes. Drain, mix with sauce, and garnish with fresh parsley and pine nuts.

TOMATO BASIL SAUCE

3-4 large tomatoes, peeled and seeded and chopped into about 1/2 inch cubes (if you want to get fancy,

if not, you can skip the peeling and seeding)

1/2 cup packed fresh basil leaves, chopped

2 garlic cloves, pressed

12-16 oz. wheat free/gluten free pasta

To easily peel tomatoes: Place tomatoes in a large bowl, pour near boiling filtered water over them and cover the bowl for 5 to 10 minutes. Peel, seed, and chop.

Pulse chop the basil and garlic in a food processor. Add the chopped tomatoes to the food processor and pulse down 5 quick times until just mixed. (Do not puree!) Pour over vegetable pasta or rice

Try adding a splash (squeeze) of lemon, plus fresh pepper.

LEMON SAUCE

(Use in "Eggs Florentine" recipe or over rice and pasta)

2 cups vegetable broth

1 1/2 Tbsp. arrowroot powder

1/4 cup lemon juice and some grated rind if it's organic

1/4 tsp. turmeric

2 Tbsp. wheat free tamari

2 garlic cloves, pressed

1/4 tsp. rice syrup or apple

or grape juice concentrate

1 1/2 Tbsp. nutritional yeast

Black pepper or cayenne to taste

Heat the broth in a heavy pot. Mix the arrowroot with about 3 Tbsp. of cold filtered water, and add it to the broth. Add the rest of the ingredients, stirring continuously until the sauce thickens.

Serve warm. Adjust the seasonings to taste. This sauce is great as a hollandaise-like sauce over vegetables, especially asparagus.

SUN DRIED TOMATO PESTO

1/3 cup pine nuts

1 Tbsp. garlic, chopped

1/3 cup fresh cilantro, packed leaves, chopped

1/3 cup fresh basil, packed leaves, chopped

1 Tbsp. lemon juice

1 cup tomato, chopped or 1/2 cup

Sun dried tomatoes in oil

1/2 tsp. sea salt

1/2 cup olive oil (preferably extra virgin, optional)

12-16 oz. wheat free/gluten free pasta

Prepare pasta as directed on the box. Put all of the ingredients into a food processor, except the tomatoes, and pulse chop several times. Stop to scrape down the sides and repeat. Add the tomatoes and continue to pulse chop until just blended. Keep a texture to the pesto; it should not be a puree. Chill or serve over rice, pasta or as a vegetable dip.

Note: Light or medium toasting of the pine nuts will add much flavor.

WHEAT FREE BREAD AND PIZZA CRUST

Servings: (2) 9x12 crusts or breads

3 cups basmati brown rice, long grain, cooked

1 small brown onion, sliced

1 garlic clove, pressed

1 tsp. wheat free tamari

1/3 cup filtered water

1 tsp. rosemary (optional)

Sauté onions and garlic in the 1/3 cup of water and the tamari. Cover for a couple of minutes until water evaporates, then stir onions and garlic into rice.

Put everything into a food processor and blend. Using wet fingers (so mixture doesn't stick to your hands) pat into a well oiled pizza pan or into a well oiled pie dish, forming a crust around perimeter. (Re-moisten fingers with water if rice gets too sticky). Bake for 15 minutes in a preheated 450° oven.

Top with pizza sauce, pesto sauce and/or your favorite vegetable pizza toppings. Bake for a few more minutes to heat the toppings. Sprinkle with nutritional yeast after it is baked for a wonderful cheesy flavor. This can also be served as it is as a flat bread. It may be easier to remove form the pan if you make several smaller crusts, about 5 or 6 inches round or square, instead of one big crust.

EGGPLANT WITH PINE NUTS AND PARSLEY

2 medium-size eggplants, or 4 small eggplants

(about 2 pounds total, stem ends cut away, sliced into 1/2 inch rounds)

Salt

Pure olive oil

2 Tbsp. pine nuts

1/4 cup chopped fresh parsley

Place the eggplant in a large colander, sprinkle liberally with salt, toss, and allow to stand for at least 30 minutes or until the eggplant begins to release its water. Dry on paper towels. Preheat the broiler.

Pour enough olive oil into a large flameproof baking pan to barely cover the bottom. One at a time, place each piece of eggplant into the pan and turn it over so that both sides are coated with oil. The eggplant slices should lie in a single layer. If you have too many pieces, cook them in two batches.

Place the pan directly under the broiler and cook until the top is evenly browned but not burned. Turn the eggplant slices over and broil again until the top is brown. Transfer to a serving dish and arrange the eggplant slices in an overlapping fashion.

Place the pine nuts in a small dry sauté pan over medium high heat. Stirring almost constantly, cook until the nuts are lightly browned, 3 to 5 minutes. Watch closely since the nuts will burn easily. Pour the nuts over the eggplant slices, sprinkle with the parsley, and serve at room temperature.

GRILLED RADICCHIO

3 small heads of radicchio

Pure olive oil

Salt

Preheat the oven broiler. Pull the outer leaves off the radicchio if they are browned or wilted, and discard. Cut the heads into quarters lengthwise from the root end. Set the radicchio pieces on a flameproof baking sheet and brush liberally with olive oil. Lightly sprinkle with salt.

Place the radicchio under the broiler, about 6 inches from the heat. Broil for about 3 to 5 minutes, or just until the top starts to brown but does not burn. Turn the oven to 500°, and bake for 10 minutes longer or until the radicchio is tender when pierced with a sharp knife. Serve hot or at room temperature.

Can also be grilled outside on a lava rock barbecue.

CUBAN BLACK BEANS

3 cups dried black beans

2 cups onions, chopped

2 cups green pepper, chopped

2 to 3 garlic cloves, minced

3 Tbsp. olive oil and 3 Tbsp. water

8 cups water

2 bay leaves

3 Tbsp. salt

3 Tbsp. onion powder

3 Tbsp. lemon juice (add before serving)

3/4 – 1 1/2 Tbsp. cumin (optional)

Cook the black beans in water until they are tender, about two hours, or use a crock pot. You may need to add more water if the beans begin to dry out. While the beans are cooking, sauté the onions, pepper and garlic in the olive oil and water. When the beans are tender, add this mixture to the beans and add the seasonings. Simmer about 30 minutes until the mixture becomes thick. Serve over rice. If you want to get fancy, garnish with chopped scallions and/or tomato wedges.

Note: If you want to save time, use pre-cooked canned beans.

SAUTÉED SPINACH AND SHIITAKE MUSHROOMS OVER RICE OR PASTA

3 Tbsp. olive oil

2 cloves garlic, minced

1/4 pound shiitake mushrooms, thinly sliced

1, 10 oz. bag fresh spinach, tough stems removed

Salt and black pepper to taste

2 cups rice or 1/2 pound wheat free/gluten free pasta

Prepare rice or pasta as directed on the box. Heat the oil in a large skillet over low heat. Add mushrooms and garlic, cover and cook about 5 minutes, stirring frequently, until the mushrooms are barely tender. Add the spinach and sprinkle lightly with salt and pepper. Cover and continue cooking for 5 to 7 minutes, stirring frequently, until the spinach is tender. Remove from the heat. Spoon over rice or pasta, or just eat it by itself.

STILL ANOTHER MARINARA SAUCE MADE WITH FRESH TOMATOES

1/2 cup extra-virgin olive oil

4 large cloves garlic, chopped

8 large ripe tomatoes, each cut into 16 wedges each, with juices

1/2 cup chopped fresh basil

Salt to taste

1 tsp. oregano

1 tsp. black pepper

12-16 oz. wheat free pasta

Prepare pasta as directed on the box. Heat the oil in a large skillet over low heat. Add the garlic and cook, stirring frequently, for 3 minutes, until golden brown. (Do not let the garlic burn). Add the tomatoes and their juices, basil, salt, and pepper. Raise the heat to medium and cover. Simmer the sauce for 10 minutes, stirring frequently, until the tomatoes are soft. Remove the cover and continue simmering for 15 minutes, until the sauce thickens slightly. Taste for seasoning.

Cook the pasta according to the package directions. Drain and turn into a serving bowl. Spoon a little sauce over the top and toss well. Spoon the remaining sauce over the top.

This is quick and easy and really impressive. Add a side salad and amaze your friends.

SPINACH PESTO

1 1/4 cups olive oil

5 large cloves garlic, chopped

4 cups packed fresh spinach, cleaned and chopped

1 Tbsp. dried basil

3 Tbsp. chopped walnuts or pine nuts

1/2 tsp. black pepper

3 Tbsp. lemon juice

Salt to taste

12-16 oz. wheat free/gluten free pasta

Prepare pasta as directed on the box. Pour the olive oil into the processor fitted with the metal small blade. Add the remaining ingredients. Process on high speed for 30 seconds, stopping 2 or 3 times to scrape down the sides with a rubber spatula. Taste for seasoning.

Note: This can be made without oil for a much lighter sauce.

BAKED EGGPLANT AND TOMATOES

2 medium eggplants, unpeeled, sliced into 3/4-inch slices

3 large tomatoes, sliced into 1/2-inch pieces

1/4 cup extra-virgin olive oil

4 cloves garlic, chopped

1/2 cup chopped fresh basil

1/2 cup chopped flat-leaf parsley

(Also called Italian parsley)

2 Tbsp. capers, rinsed

2 Tbsp. fresh rosemary leaves or 2 tsp. dried rosemary

Salt and black pepper to taste

1/3 cup hot water

Preheat the oven to 400°. In a rectangular glass baking dish, alternate slices of eggplant and tomato, overlapping, in 2 rows. Drizzle with the olive oil. Over the eggplant and tomato slices, sprinkle the garlic, basil, parsley, capers, and rosemary. Sprinkle with salt and pepper. Pour the hot water around (not on) the eggplant and tomatoes. Cover the dish tightly with foil. Bake for 45 minutes, or until the eggplant is as tender when pierced with a fork. Taste for seasoning.

Great as a main dish or over brown rice.

SPINACH BAKED MACARONI, LASAGNA OR STUFFED SHELLS

1 lb. firm tofu
1/2 tsp. salt, or more to taste
2 Tbsp. lemon juice
2 Tbsp. tahini (sesame nut butter)
1 Tbsp. olive oil
1 large onion, chopped
8 cloves garlic, pressed or minced
1/4 tsp. freshly grated nutmeg
Freshly ground black pepper to taste
8 oz. spinach leaves, finely chopped (about 8 cups loosely packed)
2 Tbsp. minced fresh basil leaves
2 Tbsp. minced fresh parsley
4 cups prepared tomato sauce
16 oz. wheat free/gluten free pasta

(This filling can also be used for lasagna or stuffed shells.) Prepare pasta as directed on the box. Blend tofu in a food processor fitted with a metal blade or a blender. Add 1/2 tsp. salt, lemon juice and tahini, blend again. Heat olive oil in a skillet over medium-high heat. Add onion; sauté about 2 minutes. Add garlic; sauté until onion is tender, about 2 minutes more. Stir in nutmeg and black pepper; sauté briefly. Stir in spinach; cook until wilted. Add basil and parsley, and remove from heat. Add sauté to processor or blender, blend with tofu mixture. Salt to taste. Mix together with cooked pasta. Preheat oven to 350°. Spread about 2 cups tomato sauce in a large glass or ceramic baking pan. Place pasta mixture in pan, spoon remaining tomato sauce on top and bake until thoroughly heated and sauce is beginning to bubble, about 30 minutes. Serve hot. This is as good as or better than any baked macaroni or lasagna you have ever had.

PEPPER AND ONION MARINARA SAUCE

3 medium onions, sliced

3 cloves garlic, chopped

2 peppers, seeded and sliced

1/4 cup vegetable oil

1 tsp. parsley flakes

1/2 tsp. sweet basil

1/2 tsp. oregano

1/4 tsp. dry mustard

1 can tomato sauce (about 40 oz.) or tomato puree

1 small (6 1/2 oz.) can tomato paste (no salt)

12 oz. mushrooms, sliced (optional)

12-16 oz. wheat free/gluten free pasta

1/2 lemon, juiced

Sauté onions, garlic, peppers and lemon in oil for about 10 minutes; add the other ingredients and simmer for about 1 hour.

Prepare pasta according to directions on box. Hint: take the juice of 1 lemon and add to the water instead of salt to make this a salt free meal.

MOM ESPOSITO'S MACARONI AND BEANS (PASTA FAGIOLI)

Servings: 6 to 8
1 (28 oz. can) Italian plum tomatoes, slightly drained and mashed
1/2 cup virgin olive oil
2 cloves garlic, minced
3/4 tsp. red pepper flakes
1/2 tsp. oregano
1 cup diced celery (preferably leaves and stalks)
1 (19 oz.) can cannellini beans
(great northern white kidney beans)
Salt to taste
12-16 oz. ditalini pasta or any small wheat free/gluten free pasta such as shells or twists

Put olive oil, garlic, red pepper flakes, oregano and celery in a Dutch oven or other heavy pot, and sauté 10 minutes until celery softens, stirring occasionally. Add tomatoes; simmer about 45 minutes. If necessary, add some of the drained tomato liquid. Add the beans and simmer 5 minutes.

Boil the pasta according to the package directions. When draining the pasta, put a receptacle under the strainer to catch some of the water; do not drain too thoroughly, leave a little water in the pasta. Combine the pasta and tomato-bean mixture; if you like the recipe moist like soup, add some of the reserved pasta water to your taste.

This recipe is very easy, fast and economical. My friends, family and I grew up on this and it is still a favorite when we all get together.

ITALIAN-STYLE LENTILS

3 cups water

1 cup lentils

2 Tbsp. oil

1 large onion

6 oz. mushrooms

1 clove garlic, crushed

1 large can tomatoes

1 Tbsp. marjoram

1 tsp. parsley and oregano

Salt and pepper

Cook lentils in water until they are tender; add more water if they begin to dry out. In a separate saucepan, heat the oil, and add the onion. Cook the onion for 3 minutes; add mushrooms and garlic; cook 2 more minutes until soft. Add roughly chopped tomatoes to pan with juices. Add seasonings. Put in lentils; bring to boil, cover and simmer for 15 minutes until most of the liquid is absorbed, but still moist. You can serve this as a side dish, over rice or wheat free/gluten free pasta or as a baked potato topping.

TOFU SPAGHETTI SAUCE

1/2 cup olive oil

2 large onions, diced

1 pound tofu, cut into cubes

1/2 pound mushrooms

1 large can tomatoes

1 green pepper, diced

Dash of pepper

1 zucchini, sliced (optional)

12-16 oz. wheat free/gluten free pasta

Prepare pasta as directed on the box. Heat oil in a good-size frying pan. Sauté onions, then add mushrooms, tofu, green pepper and zucchini and sauté a bit more. Add pepper and tomatoes. Simmer, stirring occasionally, for 1 hour. Serve over wheat free/gluten free pasta.

BASIC MARINARA SAUCE

1, 1 pound, 12 oz. can whole Italian tomatoes

7 Tbsp. olive oil

Several sprigs of parsley

4 to 5 leaves fresh basil or 1 tsp. dried

3 cloves garlic

½ tsp. red pepper

Salt and pepper to taste

½ tsp. baking soda

1 (8 oz.) can tomato sauce

12-16 oz. wheat free/gluten free pasta

Prepare pasta as directed on the box. Mash the tomatoes. Put tomatoes (mashed) and tomato sauce in frying pan. When this comes to a boil, add in baking soda. As tomatoes boil, skim off top foam. Then add parsley and basil (chopped), olive oil, salt, pepper and red pepper. Cook over medium heat for 25 minutes.

Serve over wheat free/gluten free pasta. The baking soda helps to make this sauce a little less acidic.

VEGETABLE PASTA TOPPING

2 pounds (in any combination of 2 or more) spinach,

bok choy, rapini (Italian Broccoli), broccoli florets,

collard greens, turnip greens, cleaned, washed and chopped

1 medium onion

8 oz. mushrooms

(any kind: white, portabello, etc.)

10 sun dried tomatoes in oil

4 Tbsp. olive oil

½ tsp. crushed red pepper

2 tsp. Mrs. Dash (optional)

1 clove chopped garlic

2 cups vegetable broth (or)

2 cups water and 1 Tbsp. wheat free tamari

12-16 oz. wheat free/gluten free pasta

Sauté onion, mushrooms, red pepper, garlic and Mrs. Dash in olive oil until onions are golden brown. Add vegetables and liquid in pot, cover; cook for 10 minutes.

Spoon over wheat free/gluten free pasta or rice with more thinly sliced sun dried tomatoes on top.

ALL PURPOSE PESTO

2 cloves garlic (optional)

2 cups fresh basil leaves (about 2 bunches)

1/2 cup fresh parsley leaves

2 Tbsp. pine nuts, walnuts, or pecans

1/2 cup olive oil

1/4 tsp. freshly ground pepper

1 pound wheat free/gluten free pasta

Prepare pasta as directed on the box. Fit a food processor with the metal blade or use a blender. Add the garlic cloves, and process until pureed. Add the basil and parsley, and process to chop finely. Add the nuts, and process to chop finely. With the blades turning, slowly pour in the olive oil. Add the pepper, and process until well blended, stopping the motor as needed to scrape down the sides. Taste, and adjust the seasoning.

Store refrigerated in a tightly covered container for up to 5 days or freeze for later use.

Pesto sauces are delicious on baked, steamed or mashed potatoes, on wheat free/gluten free pasta or rice, or with steamed vegetables as a dip. Any of these will make a great meal.

POLENTA AND MUSHROOMS

1 cup rice, almond or other non-dairy milk

1 to 1 1/2 Tbsp. freshly ground pepper

1 tsp. salt

1 1/4 cups instant polenta (a corn meal similar to grits often used in Italian dishes)

5 cups water

Bring 5 cups of water to a boil in a heavy medium saucepan. Add the salt. Gradually whisk in the polenta over moderate heat. Cook, stirring with a wooden spoon, until thickened and smooth, about 5 minutes. Stir the milk, salt and pepper into the polenta. Remove from the heat. Spoon the polenta onto individual plates and serve with the mushroom topping. (See recipe on next page.)

MUSHROOM TOPPING

1/2 cup dried porcini mushrooms (1/2 oz.)
4 Tbsp. olive oil
3/4 pound assorted fresh mushrooms, such as cremini and shiitake, stems trimmed (or discarded if using shiitakes), large caps quartered or thickly sliced
Salt and freshly ground pepper to taste
1 Tbsp. finely chopped shallots
1 garlic clove, minced
1/2 cup finely chopped fresh flat-leaf parsley
4 Tbsp. olive oil

In a small bowl, soak the porcinis in 1 1/2 cups of hot water until softened, about 15 minutes. Meanwhile, place 1 Tbsp. of oil in a large skillet. Add 1/3 of the fresh mushrooms; season with salt and pepper, and cook over moderately high heat, stirring occasionally, until lightly browned, about 4 minutes. Transfer to a large plate. Repeat the process twice with 2 more Tbsp. of oil and the remaining fresh mushrooms, then return all the cooked mushrooms to the pan. Drain the porcinis, reserving the soaking liquid. Rinse and coarsely chop the porcinis and add them to the pan with the shallots and garlic. Cook over moderate heat, stirring, for 3 minutes. Add the porcini liquid, stopping when you reach the grit at the bottom. Boil over high heat until reduced by half, about 4 minutes. Stir in the parsley, and season with salt and pepper. Remove from the heat, and stir in the remaining 1 Tbsp. oil. Serve at once.

CURRIED LENTILS WITH SPINACH

3 cups water

1 cup dried lentils

1 Tbsp. oil

2 cloves garlic, minced

1/2 lb. fresh spinach leaves, stemmed, washed, and chopped

28 oz. can chopped tomatoes with liquid

2 tsp. curry powder

1/2 tsp. freshly grated ginger

1/4 tsp. each of cinnamon and nutmeg

1/2 cup raisins

Wash and sort lentils, and cook until they are tender (about 1 hour), but still keep their shape. Add more water if they begin to dry out.

Heat oil in large skillet. Add the garlic and sauté over low heat for 1 minute. Add the spinach leaves; cover and steam until wilted.

Add the lentils and remaining ingredients to skillet. Cover and simmer over low heat for 20 minutes.

Serve over brown rice or mashed potatoes.

SAGE PASTA

1/2 lb. rice, corn, or quinoa elbow or twist pasta

3 Tbsp. olive oil

3 medium carrots, sliced very thin

9 scallions, cut diagonally into 1 1/2-inch pieces

40 fresh sage leaves, stems removed

Salt and pepper to taste

Juice from 1/2 lemon

Prepare pasta according to package directions. Meanwhile, heat a large skillet over medium-high heat. Add 1 1/2 Tbsp. oil. When oil is hot and sizzling, add carrots, and sauté until soft and golden, about 7 minutes. Add scallions and sage leaves to carrots. Continue to sauté until sage begins to crisp and scallions are brown, about 7 minutes. Reduce heat, and cover to keep warm. Add salt and pepper to taste.

When pasta has been cooked al dente (still a little firm) drain and return to cooking pot. Add lemon juice and remaining 1 1/2 Tbsp. oil. Toss lightly. Top with the vegetable mix and serve immediately.

ORIENTAL PATTIES

Soak overnight:
1/2 cup dry garbanzo beans (also called chick peas)
(You can often find them with the dry beans in the health food section) soaked in 2 cups water
OR
3/4 cup canned garbanzo beans (no need to soak these, they are ready to use)

Combine the following in a bowl and set aside:
1 cup very finely chopped cabbage
1/2 cup grated carrot, packed
1/2 cup minced celery
1/2 cup minced onion

Drain garbanzos.

Whiz the following in the blender until very smooth:
Soaked garbanzo beans
1/4 cup water (add enough to make mixture thick enough to shape into patties)
3/4 tsp. salt (or a little less)
1 tsp. garlic powder
3/4 tsp. dried sweet basil

Pour contents of blender into chopped vegetables and mix well.

Shape into 1/2-inch thick patties, and fry on a very lightly oiled skillet over a low to medium heat, keeping pan covered to ensure thorough cooking. These patties will be very soft but will firm up as they cool. Serve with your favorite burger toppings.

FANCY VEGGIE PASTA

VEGETABLES
1 clove garlic, minced
1 shallot, minced
1 cup basil leaves, slivered
2 cups thin asparagus
and/or snow peas and/or mushrooms
2 Tbsp. white sesame seeds
1 Tbsp. cornstarch
1 Tbsp. cold water

SAUCE
3 Tbsp. fresh lemon juice
3 Tbsp. tomato sauce
2 Tbsp. light tamari
2 Tbsp. lime juice
2 Tbsp. rice syrup or apple or grape juice concentrate
1 tsp. lime peel, grated or finely minced
1/2 tsp. Chinese chili sauce or hot sauce
Salt to taste
1/2 pound dried spaghetti-style rice or corn noodles
2 Tbsp. cooking oil

Prepare the garlic, shallot and basil. Set aside 2 cups of vegetables cut into slivers.

Place an ungreased skillet over high heat; add the sesame seeds, and toast until lightly golden. Set aside. Mix the cornstarch and cold water. Combine sauce ingredients. Set aside.

Bring at least 4 quarts of water to a vigorous boil. Lightly salt the water, and add the noodles. Cook the noodles until they lose their raw taste but are still firm, about 5 minutes. Immediately drain in a colander.

Place a 12-inch sauté pan over high heat. Add the oil, garlic, and shallots, and sauté for 15 seconds; when the garlic begins to sizzle, add the vegetables. Sauté the vegetables until they brighten, about 1 minute.

Transfer noodles to a sauté pan, and add the basil, sesame seeds, and sauce. Stir and toss, mixing the vegetables evenly with the noodles. Add the cornstarch solution, and cook until the noodles are glazed with the sauce. Taste, and adjust the seasonings, especially for salt, then serve at once or serve as a cold pasta salad.

COCONUT VEGGIE NOODLES

NOODLES

1/2 pound dried spaghetti-style noodles (corn or rice)
4 Tbsp. vegetable oil
1 cup thinly sliced fresh button mushrooms
1 sweet red pepper, seeded and slivered
1 cup slivered red cabbage
1 cup stemmed and slivered snow peas
1/4 cup chopped fresh basil
1/3 cup chopped fresh mint leaves
1/3 cup chopped green onions

SAUCE

3/4 cup unsweetened coconut milk
2 Tbsp. fresh lemon juice
2 Tbsp. wheat free/gluten free tamari
1 tsp. Chinese chili sauce or hot sauce
1/4 tsp. salt
1 Tbsp. cornstarch
1 Tbsp. cold water

Place the noodles into 4 quarts of rapidly boiling water. Cook until they lose their raw taste but are still firm, about 5 minutes. Drain; rinse with hot water, and drain again. Toss the noodles with 2 Tbsp. of the vegetable oil. Toss the vegetables and herbs with the noodles until evenly mixed. In a small bowl, combine the sauce ingredients. Combine the cornstarch with cold water, and set aside.

Place a skillet over highest heat. Add the remaining 2 Tbsp. of vegetable oil. When very hot, add the noodle mixture. Sauté for about 3 minutes until the noodles begin to heat. Add the sauce, and bring it to a low boil. Stir in a little of the cornstarch mixture, and continue cooking until the noodles are well heated. Serve at once.

MARINATED EGGPLANT

1 medium-sized eggplant, unblemished and firm
Salt
1 - 2 Tbsp. olive oil
2 Tbsp. fresh lemon juice
1 to 2 medium-sized cloves garlic, crushed
Freshly ground black pepper
Fresh marjoram, dill, and parsley,
Very finely minced

Preheat oven to 375°. Lightly oil a baking sheet. Slice eggplant into circles, about 1/2 -inch thick. Arrange the slices on the baking sheet, and salt very lightly. Let stand for about 15 to 20 minutes, then pat the eggplant dry with paper towels. Bake until the eggplant is very tender (20 to 25 minutes).

Remove the slices from the baking sheet, and place them on a large serving platter - ideally, one with a rim. The slices can be arranged in a slightly overlapping pattern.

While the eggplant is still hot, drizzle with 1 to 2 Tbsp. olive oil and the lemon juice. Spread the crushed garlic over the eggplant. Sprinkle liberally with black pepper and minced fresh herbs.

Cool to room temperature. Cover the plate very tightly with plastic wrap and chill for at least several hours, preferably overnight. Serve cold or at room temperature.

*NOTE: This takes at least 3 hours to marinate before serving, but is better if not served for 24 hours.

TOFU REUBEN SANDWICHES

1 pound extra firm tofu

6 slices dried gluten free bread ground into crumbs in a blender

8 slices fresh gluten free bread, toasted

1/2 cup non-dairy milk or water

1 cup sauerkraut

1/4 cup vegan mayonnaise

1/4 cup organic ketchup

1/4 cup organic sweet pickle relish

Oil for cooking

Black pepper

Slice tofu into 8 equal slices. Dip in milk or water, then coat with gluten free bread crumbs on both sides. In a fry pan, put enough oil to just cover the bottom and heat the oil. Place in the tofu slices and brown on both sides. Mix the mayonnaise, catsup and relish together. Spread this mixture on the bread, place the tofu on the bread and top with sauerkraut. Sprinkle pepper on top if you like and enjoy.

JEANI-ROSE'S TOFU AND RICE CROQUETTES

1/2 medium onion, chopped

1 Tbsp. olive oil

1 pound firm tofu, crumbled

1/4 cup almond butter

2 Tbsp. wheat free tamari

2 cups cooked brown rice

1/2 cup chopped parsley

1/2 tsp. dried dill weed

Sauté onion in olive oil. Blend tofu, almond butter, and tamari in a blender. In a large bowl, add all the ingredients. Form into patties and brown in a skillet with a little oil to prevent sticking.

Serve with mushroom-onion gravy.

CHILI CON CORNY

2 cups dried pinto beans

2 cups black beans

2 stalks celery, finely chopped

1 large carrot, finely chopped

1/3 cup garlic, finely chopped

2 cups onion, chopped

1 medium jalapeno pepper, finely chopped

1 medium red bell pepper, finely chopped

2 medium fresh tomatoes, chopped

4 cups fresh or frozen corn

8 oz. can tomato sauce

2 bay leaves

2 Tbsp. salt

1 tsp. black pepper

1/4 cup olive oil

2 1/2 cups bean water

1 bunch fresh cilantro

Place beans in a colander; spread them out, and remove all the rocks. Rinse well, place in a bowl, cover with water and let soak overnight. Drain and rinse well again. Place beans in a heavy large pot and cover with water at least 3 inches over the beans. Bring water to a boil, and then reduce to a very slow boil and cook until beans are tender but not mushy, about 45-60 minutes, stir occasionally. Do not let the water get below the level of the beans. Drain and save the liquid in one bowl and the beans in another. In the same pot the beans were cooked in heat the oil and add the garlic, onions and bay leaf and stir constantly about 3 minutes until golden. Add celery, carrots, pepper and jalapeno; stir for 4-6 minutes. Add tomato, tomato sauce, chili powder, salt, pepper and corn; stir well. Lower heat to medium and stir frequently for 10 minutes. Add bean cooking liquid to cover ingredients, return to high heat and boil; stir often. Lower heat to medium and simmer for 20-30 minutes. Add beans; stir, and taste for proper seasoning. Add cilantro, and serve. This freezes well for future use. Serve alone, over tofu burgers or over brown rice.

BAKED ASPARAGUS

2 pounds fresh asparagus
1/4 cup olive oil
Salt and pepper

Break off the tough bottoms of the asparagus, and wash very well. Preheat oven to 500°. Place the asparagus in a single layer in a flat cookie sheet or any flat baking dish. Pour on the oil, and coat the asparagus with the oil. Sprinkle on the salt and pepper, and bake for about 15-20 minutes until the asparagus just starts to brown, and when you pick one up it will bend but not droop.

Enjoy hot or cold.

FRIED RICE

2 cups cooked brown rice

1/2 pound firm tofu, cut into 1/4 inch cubes

1/2 cup chopped onion or

3 chopped green onions

1/2 cup peas, fresh or frozen

1 tsp. dried or fresh ginger

1 tsp. black pepper

2 Tbsp. wheat free tamari

2 Tbsp. vegetable oil

Heat oil in a wok or large fry pan. Add onions, and cook until golden brown. (If you are using fresh ginger, add it to the onion when you begin cooking). Add the rest of the ingredients, and stir fry for about 4 to 5 minutes. Serve hot.

EASY STIR FRY

6 ounces portabello or any mushroom

3 cups chopped nappa cabbage or bok choy

1 cup chopped onion or 4 chopped green onions

1/2 tsp. fresh ginger, chopped fine or grated

2 Tbsp. wheat free/gluten free tamari

2 Tbsp. sesame or any vegetable oil

Heat a wok or large fry pan with oil. Add ginger and cook for about 1 minute. Add mushrooms, and stir fry for about 3 to 4 minutes. If using regular onions, add them, and stir fry for about 2 minutes longer. Next add cabbage and tamari (and green onions if you are using them), and stir fry for about 2 more minutes. Serve plain or over brown rice.

CASHEW OR PEANUT BUTTER SAUCE

1/2 cup gluten free tamari

2 cloves garlic

1 oz. ginger, fresh

4 oz. peanut or cashew butter (Note: Must contain just nuts or nuts and oil, nothing else)

1 cup peanut oil

1/4 cup sesame oil

1/4 cup rice vinegar

1/4 cup rice syrup

1 tsp. crushed red pepper (chili flakes)

1 pound wheat free/gluten free pasta

Prepare pasta as directed on the box. Mix together tamari, garlic, peanut butter, rice vinegar, rice syrup and pepper in a food processor or blender. Separately mix sesame and peanut oil and slowly drizzle into tamari base with mixer running until it is emulsified. Serve over pasta sprinkled with black pepper if you like. This is a very rich sauce, use sparingly.

POTATO GARBANZO GNOCCHI

2 cups boiling water

2 cups mashed potato flakes

1/2 cup garbanzo flour

(dried garbanzo beans ground into a flour)

1/4 cup rice flour

1 tsp. garlic powder

1 tsp. non-alum baking powder

Pinch of cayenne or red pepper

1 tsp. smoked or regular nutritional yeast

1 tsp. salt

Oil for frying

Combine water and potato flakes. They will become firm and somewhat dry. Stir in remaining ingredients.

Drop by the tsp. into about 1/4 inch hot oil, and fry until golden brown. Another way is to drop gnocchi into boiling water, and boil until they rise to the top of the water. Serve with a tomato or pesto sauce or vegetable pasta topping.

MUSHROOM TOFU BURGERS

2 tsp. olive oil
2 tsp. minced garlic
1 small minced onion
1 cup sliced mushrooms of your choice
10 oz. Japanese-style extra firm tofu, drained and cubed
1 tsp. hot sauce of your choice
1 cup cooked rice
1 1/2 cups wheat free/gluten free bread crumbs.
(If you do not have any, take about 6 slices of wheat free/gluten free bread such as tapioca rice or millet, dry it out or toast it, and grind it in a blender or food processor.)
3/4 cup nutritional yeast, optional but well worth it.

In a medium frying pan, heat the oil, and cook garlic and onion until golden brown. Now add the mushrooms, tofu and hot sauce, and cook, stirring occasionally until liquid is evaporated.

Place this mixture and cooked rice in a food processor or blender, and mix. Be sure to scrape the sides with a spatula to get an even mix. Place this in a large bowl, and add 1 cup of wheat free/gluten free bread crumbs and nutritional yeast mix. The mixture should be dry enough to not stick to your hand. If it is too wet add more wheat free/gluten free bread crumbs. Mold into burger size patties. Either fry patties in a little oil until brown on one side, flip and brown on the other, or place about 5 inches under your oven broiler on a non-stick cookie sheet and brown each side.

Serve with ketchup, onion, mayonnaise or however you like your "burgers".

TORTILLA SANDWICHES

The Bread: Pre-made corn tortilla shells
(from just about any grocery store)

Place the shell in a hot dry frying pan for about 20 seconds on one side, flip over for another 20 seconds. Fill and roll up or lay flat. Sandwich filling (See other recipes), Nut Butter and Jam, Tomato Basil salad, Guacamole (for a real thrill, try adding alfalfa or radish sprouts), Sautéed peppers and onions, Mushroom Carrot Stir fry or whatever you like in a sandwich.

JAM

1 cup dried fruit

2 cups boiling water

Use any dried fruit preferably organic or at least one that does not have sulfites or sugar added. Try apples, cherries, peaches, figs, apricots, raisins, dates, prunes or currents. Place the fruit in the water, and let stand for one hour out of the refrigerator or overnight in the refrigerator. Drain off the water, and place in the food processor or the blender. Mix to your favorite consistency. Try adding 1 Tbsp. fruit concentrate or rice syrup if you like your jam really sweet. Store in a sealed jar in the refrigerator.

NUT BUTTERS

Place 2 to 4 cups of your favorite nuts (almond, cashew, peanut, filbert, walnut, or just about any nut) in a food processor or blender and whip until creamy. You can add 1/4 cup vegetable oil per cup of nuts to make it even creamer. (Be sure the oil is not hydrogenated.)

MUSHROOM CARROT STIR FRY

1 pound carrots, shredded

1 pound mushrooms (portabello, white or any kind you like) sliced thin

4 Tbsp. gluten free tamari

2 Tbsp. vegetable oil

Black pepper and ground ginger to taste

Place all ingredients in frying pan and cook until soft. Serve over rice or as a side dish.

SAUTÉED PEPPERS AND ONIONS

2 peppers (red and/or green and/or yellow)

1 medium onion

3 Tbsp. vegetable oil

Black pepper and rosemary to taste

Sauté peppers and onions until soft. Serve over rice or as a side dish.

CORN TORTILLA PIZZA

Sauce:

1 12 oz. can tomato paste
1 12 oz. can of water
1 Tbsp. oregano
1/2 tsp. red pepper

Mix together; if it is too thick, add more water. It should be about the consistency of slightly watery catsup.

The Crust:

6 large corn tortilla shells

Toppings:

Any or all of the following: sautéed onions, peppers, mushrooms, capers, or whatever you like on your pizza.
Nutritional yeast

Top shells with sauce and toppings, bake at 400° until sauce is warm, about 10 minutes. Top with nutritional yeast and serve.

TEX- MEX VEGETABLES

1/2 tsp. ground coriander

1/2 tsp. ground cumin

1/2 tsp. chili powder or to taste

pinch of salt

1 cup steamed diced carrots

1 cup steamed diced turnips

1 cup steamed rutabagas

1 cup steamed diced parsnips

Combine first four ingredients in a medium bowl, then add steamed vegetables into a lightly oiled baking dish. Place under broiler until vegetables are heated through, about 5 minutes.

Makes 4 servings.

SWEET LICORICE FLAVORED VEGETABLES

3 carrots, scraped and cut in quarters lengthwise

2 purple or golden beets, thickly sliced

1 large parsnip, thinly sliced

2 Tbsp. vegetable broth

or 1 Tbsp. water and 1 Tbsp. wheat free/gluten free tamari

1 Tbsp. olive oil

2 Tbsp. rice syrup

1 tsp. anise seed

1/2 tsp. each salt and white pepper

Place all ingredients in small saucepan. Cover; steam until roots are tender when pierced with knife, about 15 minutes.

Makes 4 servings.

SPRING RICE MEDLEY

3/4 cup long grain brown rice, cooked

1/4 cup wild rice, cooked

1 carrot grated, finely

1 large onion, finely chopped

1/4 cup green pepper and celery

1/2 tsp. white pepper

1/4 tsp. hot sauce

1/4 tsp. dry basil

Place all ingredients in a baking dish with a cover. Stir well. Bake covered at 350° for 1 hour and 15 minutes. Allow to set 10- 15 minutes before removing lid. Serve hot.

SPANISH RICE

1 1/2 cups brown rice, cooked

2 Tbsp. oil

1 onion, chopped finely

1 green pepper, chopped finely

1 small can tomato sauce

3 tomatoes, cube

Pepper, cumin, and chili powder to taste

In oiled frying pan, sauté onion and green pepper. Add cooked rice, tomatoes, tomato sauce and seasonings. Cook 10 more minutes, and it is ready to eat.

ANOTHER MARINARA SAUCE

1 lemon, pitted and sliced

3 medium onions, sliced

3 cloves garlic, chopped (optional)

2 peppers, seeded and sliced

1/2 cup vegetable oil

1 tsp. parsley flakes

1/4 tsp. sweet basil

1/2 tsp. oregano

1/4 tsp. dry mustard

1 can tomato sauce (about 40 oz.)

1 small (6 1/2 oz.) can tomato paste (no salt)

12 oz. mushrooms, sliced (optional)

1 pound wheat free/gluten free pasta Sauté onions, garlic, peppers and lemon oil for about 10 minutes. Liquefy in blender. Add other ingredients and simmer for about 1 hour.

Prepare pasta according to directions on box. Liquefy lemon in blender, and add to water instead of salt.

PASTA AND MUSHROOMS

MUSHROOMS

1 oz. dried porcini mushrooms

1/4 pound fresh shiitake mushrooms

1/2 pound small fresh button mushrooms

1 bunch chives, chopped

2 cloves garlic, minced (optional)

2 shallots, minced

SAUCE

1/2 cup vegetable broth

1/2 cup fresh lemon juice

2 Tbsp. green peppercorns, rinsed of brine and drained (optional)

1 Tbsp. tamari

1 Tbsp. oriental sesame oil

1/2 tsp. rice syrup

1/4 tsp. freshly ground black pepper

Salt to taste

1 Tbsp. cornstarch

Salt

1/2 pound dried spaghetti-style corn or rice noodles

6 Tbsp. olive oil

Soak the porcini mushrooms in 2 cups hot water for 1 hour; rinse, drain, and sliver. Discard the stems for the shiitake mushrooms, and sliver the caps. Cut the button mushrooms into very thin slices. Set aside the chives. Combine the garlic and shallots. In a small bowl, combine all of the sauce ingredients except salt.

Mix the cornstarch with the cold water. Bring at least 4 quarts of water to a vigorous boil. Lightly salt the water and add the noodles. Cook until they lose the raw taste but are still firm, about 5 minutes. Immediately drain in a colander.

Place a 12-inch sauté pan over high heat. Add the oil, garlic, and shallots. When the shallots sizzle, in about 15 seconds, add the mushrooms and sauté until they soften, about 5 minutes. Add the sauce, and bring to a vigorous boil.

Transfer the noodles to the sauté pan. Stir the cornstarch mixture, and then toss the noodles with the mushrooms until evenly combined, and the noodles are glazed with the sauce. Taste, and adjust seasonings, particularly for salt. Sprinkle on chives, and serve at once.

LENTIL STEW

1 cup cooked lentils

1 cup cooked rice

1 large can tomato sauce

1 small can tomato paste

1 onion, chopped

1 tsp. Italian dressing (or vinegar)

1 tsp. garlic powder or garlic salt

4 cups water

Cook all ingredients in large pot until tender (approximately 20 minutes).

LENTIL CHILI

Servings: Easily serves 8

4 cups dried lentils

6 - 7 cups water (tomato juice can be substituted

for about 2 cups water)

1, 1 pound can tomatoes, or 3 to 4 large ripe fresh tomatoes chopped

(peeling optional)

2 tsp. ground cumin

1 tsp. paprika

1/2 tsp. dried thyme (or about 2 tsp. minced fresh)

10 to 12 medium-sized cloves garlic, minced

2 medium-sized onions, finely chopped

(about 1 2/3 to 2 cups chopped)

2 tsp. salt

Lots of freshly ground black pepper

4 - 6 Tbsp. tomato paste

1 -2 Tbsp. red wine or balsamic vinegar

Crushed red pepper, to taste

OPTIONAL TOPPINGS:

A handful of toasted cashews

Minced fresh parsley and/or cilantro

Place lentils and 6 cups of water in a large pot. Bring to a boil, partially cover (mostly cover, but leave an air vent), and lower the heat to a simmer. Leave it this way for about 30 minutes, checking it every now and then to be sure it isn't cooking any faster than a gentle simmer. (You can chop the vegetables during this time).

Add tomatoes, cumin, paprika, thyme, garlic and onions. Stir, mostly cover again, and let it cook for another 45 to 60 minutes until the lentils are tender. Check the water level as it cooks, and add water or tomato juice in **1⁄4**-cup increments as needed, to prevent dryness. Stir from the bottom every 10 to 15 minutes during the cooking.

Add salt, black pepper and tomato paste. Stir, and continue to simmer slowly, partially covered, until the lentils are very soft (up to 30 minutes more). About 10 to 15 minutes before serving, add vinegar and red pepper. Adjust seasonings to taste, and serve with some or all or none of the optional toppings. This will take about **1⁄2** hour for the initial preparation: 2 hours total, including the cooking time.

REFRIED BEANS

3 cups cooked pinto or kidney beans (canned or precooked)

1 large onion, chopped

3 Tbsp. oil

9 oz. tomato paste

3 - 4 Tbsp. chili powder

Drain and mash cooked beans in a bowl. Sauté onion in oil. Add tomato paste, chili powder and mashed beans. Cook over medium heat until beans are heated through.

Try This: Mash 2 cups of the beans as above when recipe is all mixed, add the other cup for a chunkier refried bean.

GOURMET BLACK BEANS

Servings: At least 6

1 pound black beans (picked and washed)

In stainless steel 6 quart pot, put washed beans and water to 2-inch above beans; place on high burner and bring to a boil. Boil 2 minutes; turn off heat. Allow to soak for 1 hour.

Add:

2 cups water
1 carrot finely grated
1/4 cup red pepper (bell) finely chopped
1 large finely chopped onion
1/2 cup finely chopped celery
1/2 tsp. dry mustard, cumin, allspice and black pepper

Simmer for 1 1/2 hours. In the last 1/2 hour, add 1/4 cup fresh lemon juice. Serve over rice. Garnish with red pepper and green onion tops.

TOMATO/EGGPLANT BAKE

2 Tbsp. oil

1 small eggplant, peeled and cut into small pieces

1 can stewed tomatoes

1 onion, chopped finely

1 green pepper, chopped finely

Place eggplant, tomatoes, onion and green pepper in oiled baking dish. Bake at 350° until done (approximately 20 minutes).

VEGETARIAN STEW

1/2 cup corn (fresh, frozen or canned)

1/2 cup lima beans (frozen or canned)

1/2 cup potatoes (precooked or canned)

1/2 cup stewed tomatoes

1 onion, chopped

1 tsp. oregano

1/4 cup parsley, chopped

Salt and pepper to taste

Mix above in large pot. Cook over low heat until hot (about 10-15 minutes). Serve alone or on rice.

RATATOUILLE

1/4 cup oil

3 tomatoes, cubed

1 large zucchini, diced

1 small eggplant, cubed

1 large green pepper, diced

1 large onion, chopped

2 - 3 cloves garlic, minced

In large frying pan, sauté in oil the tomatoes, zucchini, eggplant, peppers, onions and garlic. Cook over low heat for 10-20 minutes. Serve over rice or gluten free bread.

ASPARAGUS AND MUSHROOM RISOTTO

1 Tbsp. olive oil

1 medium red onion, chopped

1 large red bell pepper, seeded and diced

8 oz. white button mushrooms, thickly sliced

4 oz. oyster or cremini mushrooms, thickly sliced

2 cloves garlic, minced

1 1/2 cups Arborio rice

4 cups simmering vegetable stock or hot tap water

1/2 cup fresh lemon juice

1 1/2 Tbsp. dried parsley or 3 to 4 Tbsp.

chopped fresh parsley

1/2 tsp. each salt and white pepper

10 to 12 asparagus spears, trimmed and cut into 1-inch pieces

In a large saucepan, heat oil over medium heat. Add onion, bell pepper, mushrooms and garlic. Cook about 8 minutes, stirring frequently. Stir in rice, 2 cups stock or water, parsley, salt and white pepper; bring to simmer over medium-high heat. Cook over low heat, uncovered, for about 10 minutes, stirring frequently.

Stir in remaining stock or water and asparagus. Cook, continuing to stir, until rice is tender, about 10 to 12 minutes. Serve hot.

ANOTHER ALFREDO SAUCE

1½ cups frozen corn kernels

1½ cups non-dairy milk

2 Tbsp. tahini (sesame seed butter)

1 Tbsp. onion granules

1 tsp. salt

Black pepper

12-16 oz. wheat free/gluten free pasta

Prepare pasta as directed on the box. Thaw corn kernels. Place the corn, milk, tahini, and seasonings in a blender, and process until completely smooth. (It may take several minutes to completely pulverize the corn). Pour the blended mixture into a medium saucepan, and warm over medium-low heat, stirring often.

While the sauce is heating, cook the pasta in a large pot of boiling water until al dente (still a little firm). Drain well, and return to the pot. Add the hot sauce, and toss until evenly coated. Serve immediately, topping each portion with pepper, if desired.

BAKED PEAS AND POTATOES

1 pound frozen or fresh peas

4 to 6 potatoes

1 1/2 cup crushed canned tomatoes

1/2 cup olive oil

1/2 tsp. oregano

1 tsp. garlic powder

1/2 tsp. hot pepper flakes

Salt and pepper

Mix all but potatoes and peas. Peel and quarter the potatoes; add to mix. Remove potatoes with your hand; place in a single layer in an oiled roasting pan. Add peas to mixture, and pour the whole mixture on top of potatoes; spread out evenly. Bake 350° for 1 hour or until potatoes are done and liquid is a little evaporated.

SUNDRIED TOMATOES AND BEANS

1 1/2 cups sun-dried tomatoes (not oil-packed)

1 Tbsp. olive oil

1 large yellow onion, dice

2 - 3 cloves garlic, minced

3 15 oz. cans cannellini beans, (or Great Northern

Beans or white kidney beans) rinsed and drained

1/4 cup water

1/2 tsp. ground sage

1/2 tsp. each salt and freshly ground black pepper

1/4 tsp. dried red pepper flakes

1/3 cup chopped fresh basil

In a small bowl, soak tomatoes in enough warm water to cover until soft, about 1 hour. Drain; coarsely chop.

In a saucepan, heat oil over medium-high heat. Add onion and garlic; cook, stirring, until onion is soft and translucent, about 4 minutes. Add beans, tomatoes, water, sage, salt, black pepper and red pepper flakes; cook for 10 to 15 minutes. Stir in basil; remove from heat. Keep warm until ready to serve.

FETTUCCINE ALFREDO

½ cup blanched almonds

½ cup water

½ cup non-dairy milk

1 minced shallot

2 cloves minced garlic

1 Tbsp. olive oil

Dash nutmeg

Salt and white pepper to taste

12-16 oz. wheat free/gluten free pasta

Prepare pasta as directed on the box. In blender or food processor, puree almonds, water and milk until smooth.

In sauté pan, cook shallot and garlic in oil on low heat until soft, about 3 minutes. Do not brown. Add almond mixture; simmer until sauce thickens, about 3 to 4 minutes. Add nutmeg, salt and pepper.

VEGETARIAN CHILI

1/4 cup oil

1 large onion, chopped

3 cloves garlic, minced

1 large green pepper, diced

3 cups water

1 cup kidney beans (precooked or canned)

4 tomatoes, cubed

1 cup corn (fresh or frozen) optional

1 tsp. salt

1 tsp. chili powder

Pepper to taste

In large pot, sauté in oil the onion, garlic and green pepper until the onion is soft. Add water, kidney beans, tomatoes, corn, salt, chili powder and pepper. Cook 25 minutes.

Try this: Add hot peppers or other vegetables such as carrots and celery. Pinto beans may be used instead of kidney beans.

PECAN PESTO

1½ cup basil leaves

⅓ cup pecans, finely ground

1 Tbsp. garlic, chopped

2-3 Tbsp. lemon juice

Pinch sea salt

1 cup olive oil (preferably virgin, optional)

1 pound wheat free/gluten free pasta

Prepare pasta as directed on the box. Rinse and tear the basil leaves in half. Put all of the ingredients into a blender and grind. You may need to stop and stir a couple of times during blending. Refrigerate the pesto if you want to use it at a later date or serve right away. Use over pasta or on baked potatoes.

EGGPLANT PASTA OR RICE SAUCE

1 eggplant

1 onion

2 garlic cloves

1/4 cup red vinegar

28 oz. can tomatoes, crushed

6 oz. can tomato paste and filtered water to thin

1 tsp. (each) oregano and basil

1/2 tsp. (each) crushed red pepper and fennel seeds

1/2 tsp. sea salt

1 Tbsp. lemon juice or 1 lemon wedge

12-16 oz. wheat free/gluten free pasta OR

2 cups brown rice

Prepare rice or pasta as directed on the box. Skin and dice the eggplant, chop the onion. Sauté the garlic in a deep skillet with vinegar. Add the eggplant and onion; continue stirring for 5 minutes or so. Add tomatoes, paste, water and rest of ingredients. Cook on low heat, covered for 1 1/2 hours. Stir occasionally. Serve over rice or pasta.

GRILLED EGGPLANT WITH SUN-DRIED TOMATOES

2 medium-size eggplants (about 1 pound each), stem ends cut away, cut lengthwise or crosswise into 1-inch thick slices

Salt

12 oil-packed sun-dried tomato halves

2 Tbsp. of the oil from the tomatoes

8 sprigs fresh parsley, washed and dried well

1/2 cup pure olive oil or more as needed for basting the eggplants

Place the eggplant slices in a colander; sprinkle liberally with salt, toss and leave them to drain for at least 30 minutes, or until the eggplants begin to release their water.

Meanwhile, combine the tomatoes, the tomato oil and the parsley in a food processor. Process for about 30 seconds or until the mixture forms a coarse paste. If you are chopping by hand, finely chop the tomatoes and the parsley separately and combine with the oil in a small bowl. Set aside. Preheat the broiler in your oven.

Dry the eggplant slices with paper towels, and arrange them in a single layer in a greased, flameproof baking dish (do not use glass because it will break under the broiler). Brush the eggplant with the olive oil. Place the pan directly under the broiler. Broil for about 5 minutes or until the eggplant begins to brown. Turn the slices over with a spatula; brush with more olive oil, and return the pan to the broiler. Cook for another 5 minutes or until the tops begin to brown.

Remove the pan from the oven, and turn off the broiler. Set the oven to bake at 325°.

Using a teaspoon, spread some of the tomato-and-parsley mixture over each slice of eggplant. The slices need only a thin covering - if you put too much on, the saltiness of the tomatoes will be overpowering.

Return the pan to the oven, and bake for 30 minutes. Transfer the eggplant slices to a serving dish and serve at room temperature.

ROOT VEGETABLES

2 turnips
3 carrots
2 sweet potatoes
1 white potato
1 onion
8 mushrooms
1 bell pepper
1 rutabaga
2 parsnips
1/3 bunch cilantro (chopped)
salt and pepper to taste
1/4 cup olive oil

Coat vegetables with oil, and bake about 1 hour or until vegetables are cooked. Serve hot.

SWISS CHARD ITALIAN STYLE

1 bunch Swiss chard

1 16 oz. can stewed tomatoes

1 medium onion, chopped fine

1 clove garlic, chopped fine

Parboil Swiss chard for 15 minutes; drain all water off and chop. Sauté onion and garlic in oil until soft, then add stewed tomatoes, then put back Swiss chard with onions, garlic and tomatoes; cook 15 minutes. This is a quick side dish or a main course with a few slices of wheat free/gluten free bread.

BAKED RED PEPPERS

6 to 8 red peppers

5 garlic cloves

2 oz. capers

Black olives

Black pepper

1/2 cup red vinegar

1/4 cup olive oil

Slice peppers in strips; cut up garlic. Add capers and sliced olives. Add black pepper, vinegar and oil. Place all ingredients in baking pan; cover with aluminum foil. Bake 15 minutes at 350°. Uncover, stir and put back in oven for 15 minutes. This will impress your guests when served as a snack food with wheat free crackers, or as a warm or cold salad.

FANCY VEGGIE PASTA

VEGETABLES

1 clove garlic, minced

1 shallot, minced

1 cup basil leaves, slivered

2 cups thin asparagus and/or snow peas and/or mushrooms

2 Tbsp. white sesame seeds

1 Tbsp. cornstarch

1 Tbsp. cold water

SAUCE

3 Tbsp. fresh lemon juice

3 Tbsp. tomato sauce

2 Tbsp. light wheat free/gluten free tamari

2 Tbsp. lime juice

2 Tbsp. rice syrup or apple or grape juice concentrate

1 tsp. lime peel, grated or finely minced

1/2 tsp. Chinese chili sauce or hot sauce

Salt to taste

1/2 pound wheat free spaghetti-style pasta

2 Tbsp. cooking oil

Prepare the garlic, shallot and basil. Set aside 2 cups of vegetables; cut into slivers.

Place an ungreased skillet over high heat; add the sesame seeds, and toast until lightly golden. Set aside. Mix the cornstarch and cold water. Combine sauce ingredients. Set aside.

Bring at least 4 quarts of water to a vigorous boil. Lightly salt the water, and add the noodles. Cook the noodles until they lose their raw taste but are still firm, about 5 minutes. Immediately drain in a colander.

Place a 12-inch sauté pan over high heat. Add the oil, garlic, and shallots, and sauté for 15 seconds; when the garlic begins to sizzle, add the vegetables. Sauté the vegetables until they brighten, about 1 minute.

Transfer noodles to a sauté pan, and add the basil, sesame seeds and sauce. Stir and toss, mixing the vegetables evenly with the noodles. Add the cornstarch solution, and cook until the noodles are glazed with the sauce. Taste, and adjust the seasonings, especially for salt, then serve at once or serve as a cold pasta salad.

SWEET AND SOUR VEGGIES

1 small head cabbage

3 large yellow squash

2 medium sweet potatoes

4 stalks celery

3 carrots

1 large onion

1 green pepper

1/4 cup orange juice

1/4 cup rice syrup or apple or grape juice concentrate

1 10 oz. can pineapple chunks

1/4 cup apple cider vinegar

1 tsp. salt

Chop all vegetables and place in large pot. Add pineapple with juice, orange juice and rice syrup. Simmer one hour over medium heat, adding water as needed. Stir in vinegar and salt. Serve over rice, if desired.

BRAISED ARTICHOKES

4 artichokes, fresh

Olive oil

1 clove garlic

6 sprigs Italian parsley

black pepper and salt

1/4 cup red vinegar

<u>Cleaning the artichoke:</u>

Slice bottom stem off, and save a few of the remaining outer leaves. Lay artichoke on its side, and slice off the top of the artichoke, about 1/4 of it, to remove the sharp points on the top of the leaves. Hold artichoke by the bottom, and hit the top gently against the counter; this will spread the leaves open. Wash thoroughly in running water; drain water out by placing upside down.

Peel and dice stem you cut off; mince garlic and parsley. Add black pepper, salt and 2 Tbsp. olive oil, and mix. Stuff mix in artichoke between leaves with a tsp.; sprinkle any remaining mix on top. Use a heavy bottom pot that will hold artichokes up right and next to each other.

Put a thin film of oil in pot; add artichokes vinegar and water to cover 1/2 of artichokes. Cover and steam about 30 minutes to 1 hour. To test for doneness, pull out a leaf, and taste (hold by top and pull leaf through your teeth), it should be soft, if not, cook until tender. The water will evaporate, and the artichokes will brown on the bottom. If the artichokes start to burn and are still not done, just add more water and continue to steam. Eat the bottom but do not eat the fuzzy part in the middle. Remove with a knife or spoon.

These are what I call a fun food - they are messy and delicious, and just fun to eat.

CARROTS, TURNIPS AND RUTABAGAS

1 large or 2 medium rutabagas

2 large carrots, quartered

1 medium turnip, quartered

1/4 cup vegetable broth

1 Tbsp. apple juice concentrate

1 Tbsp. rice syrup

1 tsp. grated lemon rind, organic

Preheat oven to 350°. Lightly oil 2 quart casserole dish. Arrange carrots, turnips and rutabagas in the dish. In a small bowl combine apple juice concentrate, rice syrup and lemon rind. Drizzle over vegetables and cover with foil. Bake until tender, about 50 minutes.

MILLET LOAF

1 cup dried millet

5 cups tomato juice

1 medium onion, chopped

1 cup raw cashews, chopped finely

1 can chopped black olives

1 tsp. dried sage

1 tsp. dried savory

1 tsp. salt

Mix all ingredients, and bake in a shallow baking dish covered at 325° for 3 to 3½ hours or until liquid is absorbed and millet is soft. Bake an additional ½ hour uncovered. Slice and serve as is or with a brown gravy.

Plenty of Potato Preparations

LEFTOVER POTATO DISH

2 cups leftover baked or boiled potatoes, sliced

1 onion, chopped

1 cup leftover cooked vegetables

1/4 cup oil

Paprika, garlic salt and pepper to taste

In large oiled frying pan, fry potatoes and onions. Add vegetables and seasoning. Heat 5 minutes.

BAKED FRENCH FRIES

Potatoes, preferably organic

Olive oil (optional)

Preheat the oven to 450°.Scrub the potatoes. Slice them into the desired size and shape. Place the "fries" on a cookie sheet. Bake 30 to 40 minutes, depending on size of the potato slices. Brush the potatoes with a little olive oil to give them a fried flavor, but this is not necessary.

Try this with garlic powder and/or paprika, shiitake mushroom gravy, mushroom sage gravy or tofu mayonnaise.

TINY STUFFED POTATOES

Servings: 10 to 12 as an appetizer, 6 to 8 as a side dish

POTATOES
1 1/2 pounds small new red potatoes, 12-16,
unpeeled and well scrubbed
2 Tbsp. olive oil

FILLING
2 Tbsp. olive oil
1 small yellow onion, finely chopped
1 globe eggplant, 1 1/2 -2 pounds peeled and cut into 1/8" dice
2 red bell peppers seeded, and cut into 1/8" dice
2 pounds plum (Roma) tomatoes, peeled, seeded and finely chopped
2 cloves garlic, minced
2 Tbsp. finely chopped fresh basil
1 Tbsp. balsamic vinegar
1 tsp. salt
1/4 tsp. freshly ground pepper

Preheat an oven to 475°. Bake potatoes first by placing the potatoes on a baking sheet in the middle of the oven. Bake until tender and slightly crispy, 45-50 minutes; test with a knife or fork. Remove and let cool. Leave the oven set on.

Cut each potato in half. If the ends are uneven, cut off a thin slice so they will stand upright once filled. Scoop out the pulp from each half, leaving only a thin shell of pulp; reserve the pulp for another use. Return the potato shells to the baking sheet, hollow sides down, and brush the skins with olive oil. Bake until crisp, 10-15 minutes. Remove from the oven, and reduce the oven temperature to 425°.

While the potatoes are cooling, make the stuffing. In a large frying pan over medium heat, warm the olive oil. Add the onion and sauté, stirring frequently, until translucent, about 5 minutes. Add the eggplant and cook, stirring, until beginning to soften, 5- 7 minutes. Add the bell peppers and cook, stirring, 5 minutes longer. Add the tomatoes, garlic, basil and vinegar; continue cooking until the liquid evaporates and the eggplant is soft, about 5-10 minutes longer. Season with the salt and pepper. Set aside.

Spoon in the filling, and place on an ungreased baking sheet. Bake until heated through, 10-15 minutes. Serve immediately.

HOME FRIES

Serving: 2 potatoes per person, baked or steamed, and cooled

1 Tbsp. olive oil per potato (optional)

Paprika

Rosemary

Black and/or white pepper

Scrub potatoes well, and slice the potatoes into 1/4 inch slices. Place them in a non-stick pan over medium heat with oil if you prefer. Sprinkle with any or all seasonings. Turn the "fries" with a spatula every 5 minutes until the potatoes are a golden brown. If the potatoes are not browning, let them sit a little longer between the turnings. Before serving, sprinkle with dried herbs and paprika.

POTATO PANCAKES

3 potatoes, cleaned and shredded

2 cups cooked brown rice

3 Tbsp. scallions, minced

1 tsp. garlic powder

1 cup brown rice flour

Combine all the ingredients in a large mixing bowl. Mix well. With a large spoon or by hand, scoop out approximately 1/2 cup of the mix at a time. Shape the mix into 3"diameter pancakes. Continue until batter is finished.

In a heated, non-stick skillet, over medium-low heat, place as many cakes as possible. Make sure all cakes are flat in the pan. Cook 25 minutes. Check to be sure they are not burning. Turn and cook an additional 25 minutes. Remove from pan, and start another batch. Reserve prepared cakes in warm oven.

Short Cut: Mix all the ingredients in a mixing bowl. Mix well. Transfer to a 9"x 13"baking dish, and cook covered in 375° oven for 45 minutes, and cut into squares and serve plain or with vegetarian sour cream and/or apple sauce.

BARBECUE POTATOES AND SUN DRIED TOMATO PESTO

18 small new red potatoes, about 1 3⁄4 lb., unpeeled
and well scrubbed
Salt
2 Tbsp. sun-dried tomato pesto

Fill a large pot three-fourths full with water, and bring to a boil over high heat. Add salt to taste and the potatoes, and cook for 10 minutes. Drain well in a colander, and set aside to cool.

Meanwhile, prepare a lava rock barbecue.

Oil six 6-inch square of aluminum foil. Arrange 3 potatoes on the center of each foil square. Spoon 1 tsp. of the pesto atop each portion of potatoes. Enclose the potatoes in the foil and seal tightly closed.

Place the foil packages on the grill rack about 3 inches from the fire and grill, turning once, until the potatoes are cooked through, 6-8 minutes per side.

Transfer the potato packages to a serving platter. Serve immediately, opening each package carefully with potholder-protected hands just before serving.

ROASTED POTATOES - CAJUN STYLE

2½ pounds yellow-fleshed, red or white potatoes (5 or 6 potatoes, preferably organic)

¼ cup vegetable oil or olive oil

2 shallots, finely chopped

1 clove garlic, minced

1 tsp. salt

½ tsp. paprika

½ tsp. cayenne pepper

½ tsp. freshly ground black pepper

2 Tbsp. chopped fresh parsley, use to garnish

Preheat an oven to 450°, scrub potatoes really well under cold water, then rinse under cold running water, and pat dry with a kitchen towel. Cut each potato lengthwise into 8 wedges.

In a roasting pan stir together the oil, shallots, garlic, salt, paprika, cayenne pepper and black pepper. Add the potatoes and, using a pancake flipper or by shaking the pan from side to side or using your hands, coat them evenly with the oil mixture. Place in oven, turning them every 15 minutes, until golden brown, about 45 minutes. Taste, and adjust the seasoning.

Garnish with parsley and serve.

PESTO POTATO WEDGES

2 basic baked potatoes, hot

3 Tbsp. pesto (see other recipes)

Preheat a broiler (griller). Cut each potato in half lengthwise and then in half again, to create 4 wedges. Spread the cut sides of each wedge evenly with some of the pesto, and place the wedges on an ungreased baking sheet, pesto side up. Place under the broiler; broil (grill) until bubbling, about 3 minutes. Serve immediately.

POTATOES WITH LEMON, BASIL AND CHIVES

2 1/2 pounds new red or white potatoes, unpeeled

1/4 cup olive oil

2 Tbsp. fresh lemon juice

1 tsp. salt

1/4 tsp. paprika

1/2 tsp. freshly ground pepper

1 Tbsp. finely chopped fresh basil

1 Tbsp. finely chopped fresh chives

Preheat an oven to 425°. Scrub potatoes under cold running water, and pat dry with a kitchen towel. In a roasting pan, mix together the olive oil, lemon juice, salt, paprika, and pepper. Add the potatoes and, using a pancake flipper or by shaking the pan from side to side or using your hands, coat the potatoes evenly with the oil mixture. Roast the potatoes, turning every 15 minutes, until golden brown, about 45 minutes. Taste, and adjust the seasoning.

Garnish with the basil and enjoy!!!

Soup-er Recipes

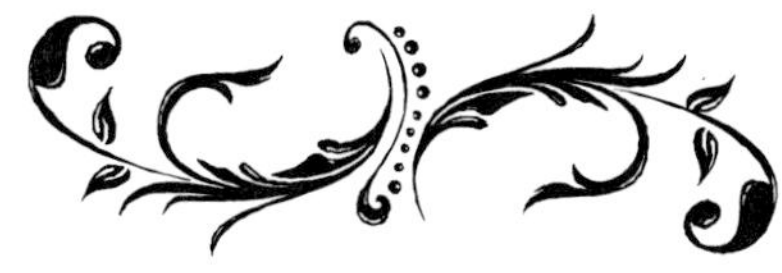

BASIC VEGETABLE BROTH

1 pot of filtered or distilled water (2 quarts)

3 cups greens, packed (beet, chard, etc.)

1 carrot top and leaves

1 cup fresh parsley

1 onion, peeled and chopped

Bring the water to a boil; add the vegetables, then simmer them for 15-30 minutes on low. Turn the heat off, and keep the stock covered overnight. Strain broth in the morning (discard the vegetables). The broth can be used fresh or frozen for later use. Be sure to freeze it in amounts that are easy to use.

HOT AND SOUR SOUP

4 cups each vegetable broth and water

8 mushrooms, diced

1 red bell pepper, diced

1 carrot, sliced diagonally

1 large onion, diced

1 clove garlic, minced

1 dozen snow peas, quartered diagonally

14 oz. firm tofu, diced

1/4 cup each, gluten free tamari sauce, and vinegar

1/2 cup cornstarch

1/2 tsp. each, black pepper, red pepper, flaked white pepper, and sesame oil

6 green onions, sliced diagonally

1/4 cup chopped cilantro

In a large pot over high heat bring broth and water to a boil. Stir in mushrooms, bell pepper, carrot, onion and garlic; return to a boil once again.

In a small bowl, stir together tamari sauce, vinegar, cornstarch, pepper, sesame oil and red pepper flakes. Stirring briskly, add cornstarch mixture to bubbling soup. When mixture has come to a full boil and is thickened and clear, stir in cilantro and green onions. Makes 8 servings.

LIMA BEAN CORN CHOWDER

2 cups dry lima beans

4½ cups water

1 onion, chopped

3 celery stalks, chopped

2 Tbsp. vegetable oil

1 tsp. dried basil

½ tsp. dried thyme

1 tsp. garlic powder

Salt and freshly ground black pepper to taste

4 cups frozen corn kernels

¼ cup tamari

1 cup non-dairy milk

Cook lima beans in water until tender, about 1 hour. Set lima beans aside, reserving cooking liquid.

In sauté pan over medium-low heat, cook onion, celery and dry seasonings in oil until onion is soft about 5 minutes. In food processor or blender, puree half of lima beans with cooking liquid. Add puree and onion-corn mixture to remaining limas and cooking liquid. Bring mixture to simmer. Add tamari and milk. Heat to serving temperature, but do not boil. If too thick, add more cooking liquid or water. Makes 10 servings.

ASPARAGUS/LEEK SOUP

1½ pounds leeks (4-6 leeks)

4 medium onions

2 medium potatoes

3 cups water

4⅔ cups vegetable stock

2 bunches asparagus (trimmed and blanched)

4 Tbsp. olive oil

2½ Tbsp. snipped chives

Salt, white pepper, and garlic to taste

Trim, wash and chop leeks, using only the white parts (reserve the green parts for stock). Peel, wash and slice onions (fine). Peel potatoes, and cut them into large, even chunks. Trim and blanch asparagus (reserve trimmings for stock).

Heat olive oil in a saucepan, and gently sauté leeks and onions. Add water and stock. Add potatoes, and simmer 20 minutes (time may vary). Pureé mixture in blender or processor, and rub through a sieve into a holding pan or bowl. Season to taste. Add asparagus spears and chives to garnish.

Serve cold (like vichyssoise)

TROPICAL BRISQUE

3 cups papaya flesh, chopped

1/2 cup coconut milk (or lite almond milk with 1/2 tsp. coconut extract)

5 Tbsp. chopped dates, pitted

1/4 cup lime juice, fresh

1 cup filtered water

1/4 cup orange juice

7 mint leaves, chopped

Blend all of the ingredients until smooth and creamy. Chill before serving; garnish each bowl with a mint leaf.

CARROT SOUP WITH CILANTRO

1 Tbsp. vegetable oil

1/2 tsp. fennel seeds

1 apple, peeled, cored and diced

1 1/2 pounds carrots, sliced

1/2 pound sweet potatoes or yams, peeled and cubed

2 Tbsp. white or brown basmati rice

or regular long-grain rice

1/4 tsp. turmeric or curry powder

5 1/2 cups vegetable stock or 5 1/2 cups water and 4 Tbsp. wheat free/gluten free tamari

1 bay leaf

Salt, pepper and lemon juice to taste

2 Tbsp. minced cilantro or parsley

Warm oil in a soup pot over medium heat. Add fennel seeds and toast until darkened, about 2 to 3 minutes. Add apple, carrots, sweet potatoes or yams; cook about 5 minutes, stirring occasionally. Add rice, turmeric or curry powder, vegetable stock or water and bay leaf.

Bring to a boil; reduce heat. Cover and simmer until rice is done, and vegetables are tender, about 30 minutes. Discard bay leaf. Transfer vegetables and small amounts of broth in batches to food processor or blender, and puree until smooth. Return pureed soup to soup pot. Simmer for about 5 minutes. Season with salt, pepper and lemon juice if desired. Enjoy!!!

GAZPACHO SOUP

2 cups tomato juice

2 Tbsp. lemon juice

1 Tbsp. salt

1 small garlic clove

2 Tbsp. olive oil

Pour above mixture into a bowl and add:

1 cup chopped tomatoes

1/2 cup chopped green peppers

1/2 cup chopped cucumber

2 Tbsp. chopped parsley (fresh)

1/2 cup chopped celery

1/4 cup chopped onion

1 Tbsp. chopped chives (scallion tops may be used in place of chives)

Chill and serve.

SPINACH, ESCAROLE, AND RICE SOUP

4 Tbsp. olive oil

1 small onion, finely chopped

1, 10 oz. package fresh spinach, stems removed and thoroughly washed, or one 10 oz. package frozen chopped spinach, defrosted

1 bunch escarole, roughly chopped

4 cups vegetable broth or water

1/2 cup uncooked short-grain Italian rice, preferably

Arborio, however any rice will do

Salt and freshly ground black pepper to taste

Melt the butter in a medium-size flameproof casserole or large saucepan over medium-high heat. Add the onion and cook, stirring, for 2 to 3 minutes, until the onion begins to soften. Add the spinach and cook, stirring, for about 5 minutes, until the spinach is wilted or, if you are using frozen spinach, heated through. Stir in the escarole and cook for 3 to 5 minutes, until soft. Add the broth, turn the heat to high and bring the soup to a boil. Add the rice, lower the heat to medium and cook, covered, for 20 minutes, or until the rice is tender but still firm.

Season with salt and pepper; ladle into bowls, and enjoy.

LIMA BEAN SOUP

1 cup vegetable stock

1 (20 oz.) bag frozen lima beans, defrosted

1½ stalks celery without leaves, sliced

2 medium carrots, sliced

1 medium tomato, chopped

1 medium onion, chopped

1 leek (white part only), sliced

3 cloves garlic, chopped

1 medium bay leaf, broken in half

½ tsp. each sage, basil and thyme, crushed

2 Tbsp. Italian flat leaf parsley, chopped

2 Tbsp. tamari

Combine all ingredients except parsley in a large pot, and bring to a boil. Reduce heat, and simmer until vegetables are tender, about 30 minutes. Serve hot, and garnish with parsley.

TOMATO BUTTERNUT SOUP

1 medium butternut squash (or any winter squash), peeled and diced

2 cups non-dairy milk

2, 14.5 oz. can diced tomatoes

1-2 tsp. salt to taste

1 Tbsp. fresh ginger (optional)

Place squash in saucepan with milk. Simmer until squash is soft. Add 1 can of diced tomatoes, and puree with squash. Add second can of diced tomatoes, leaving in chunks. Heat, add salt and ginger, then serve. Garnish with green onions. Delicious and easy!

TOMATO & RICE SOUP

1 small onion, chopped

2 garlic cloves, crushed

1 (1 lb., 12 oz.) can tomatoes

2 Tbsp. tomato paste

1 Tbsp. chopped fresh basil or 1/2 tsp. dried leaf basil

2 1/2 cups water

4 Tbsp. apple juice

1/3 cup cooked long grain Basmati Rice

Salt and pepper to taste

Fresh basil leaves to garnish

2 Tbsp. vinegar

In a large saucepan, combine onion, garlic, tomatoes with juice, tomato paste, chopped basil and water. Bring to a boil, cover and simmer 30 minutes. In a food processor fitted with a metal blade or a blender, process tomato mixture to a puree. Clean pan. Pour puree through a sieve set over a clean pan.

Return to a boil and add rice. Reduce heat, and simmer 15 minutes or until rice is tender. Season with salt, vinegar and pepper. Garnish with basil leaves.

CREAMY CARROT SOUP

2 Tbsp. olive oil

1 small onion, finely chopped

1 medium-size potato, diced

1 pound carrots, chopped

3 cups vegetable stock (canned, mixed from powder or homemade)

1 Tbsp. rice syrup or apple or grape juice concentrate

2/3 cup coconut or any nut milk

Salt and pepper to taste

Pour oil in a large saucepan. Add onion, potato and carrots. Cover and cook over low heat 10 minutes. Add stock and sweetener. Bring to a boil, and then simmer 30 minutes. In a food processor fitted with a metal blade or a blender, process mixture to a puree. Clean pan and return puree to clean pan. Stir in milk and season with salt and pepper.

FANCY VEGETABLE BROTH

1 small onion, thinly sliced

1 leek, chopped

2 stalks celery, chopped

3 carrots, chopped

2 tomatoes, chopped

5 cups water

1 Bouquet garni (a fancy way of saying 3-4 dried Tbsp. of your favorite herbs - such as rosemary, thyme, oregano, basil, etc. tied up in a cheese cloth)

2 bay leaves

Salt to taste

½ tsp. black peppercorns

To prepare stock, combine all stock ingredients in a large saucepan. Bring to a boil, and simmer 40 minutes. For a stronger flavor, boil rapidly 5 minutes or until stock is reduced to 3¾ cups. Strain stock into a large bowl.

EASY VEGETABLE SOUP

2 carrots, thinly sliced

2 stalks celery, sliced

2 oz. button mushrooms, sliced

1 1/4 cups broccoli florets (tops)

1/2 cup frozen green peas

1 zucchini cut in strips

salt and pepper to taste

Fresh flat-leaf parsley sprigs to garnish

3-4 cups vegetable broth

Place broth into a sauce pan. Add carrots, celery, mushrooms and broccoli. Bring to a boil. Cover and simmer 5 minutes. Stir in green peas and zucchini and cook 2 minutes. Season with salt and pepper. Garnish with parsley sprigs.

VEGETABLE SOUP ANOTHER WAY

12 oz. carrots, chopped

8 oz. rutabagas, chopped

2 small leeks, chopped

4 oz. potatoes, diced

3 3/4 cups vegetable broth

1 1/4 cups coconut milk or any nut milk

salt and pepper to taste

1 Tbsp. chopped fresh parsley

Additional chopped fresh parsley to garnish, if desired

In a large saucepan, combine all vegetables and stock. Bring to a boil. Cover and simmer 30 minutes. Stir in milk. Reheat and season with salt and pepper.

CURRIED SQUASH AND TURNIP SOUP

4 cups water

3 small to medium turnip roots

1 large butternut squash

2 tsp. sea salt

1/2 tsp. wheat free tamari

1/2 tsp. white pepper

1/2 tsp. ginger (powdered)

1 tsp. curry

1 large onion

3 Tbsp. olive oil

1 1/2 tsp. prepared garlic

Peel and cube squash and turnips (1 x 1 inch cubes). In a 4 quart stock pot, add water, salt, squash and turnips; cover and cook on medium until tender.

Sauté onions, garlic and spices in oil until they get soft and clear looking.

When squash and turnips are cooked, remove them with a large slotted spoon, leaving the liquid in the pot. Puree them in a food processor or blender until smooth.

Add onion mixture to the liquid, then whisk in the squash and turnips. Cook on low for about 10 minutes. Garnish with paprika and/or parsley. Can be served hot or cold.

*For a spicier soup, increase white pepper to 1 tsp. and the curry to 1 1/2 tsp.

DILLED POTATO SOUP

Combine the following in a saucepan and cook until vegetables are tender, stirring occasionally:

4 cups potatoes, peeled and diced (1/2 inch dices)

2 cups water

1 cup finely chopped onion

1/2 cup finely chopped celery

1 1/4 tsp. salt

Then remove 1 cup of cooked vegetables from pot. Place in a bowl and mash thoroughly with:

1 tsp. dill weed (dried)

1/2 tsp. garlic powder

2 tsp. dry parsley

Return mashed ingredients to the pot, and mix in well.

Serve immediately.

GUMBO

Combine the following in a saucepan and bring to a boil:

1 cup chopped onion

2 to 3 cloves garlic, minced

½ cup chopped bell pepper

½ cup water

When boiling, add the following and continue cooking until okra is tender.

1 10-oz. package frozen cut okra (about 2 to 3 cups)

Then mix in:

1 16-oz. can tomatoes, cut in bite-sized pieces

1½ tsp. dry parsley

1 tsp. salt

1 tsp. lemon juice (helps cut the slime from the okra)

¼ tsp. sweet basil (dried)

¼ tsp. oregano

Heat thoroughly and serve.

WHITE BEAN WITH SWISS CHARD

1 cup dried white beans

8 cups water

1 bay leaf

1 medium onion

1/2 cup chopped celery

1 Tbsp. olive oil

Water or vegetable stock (optional)

3/4 tsp. salt or to taste

2 to 3 Tbsp. red vinegar

One quart washed and chopped Swiss chard leaves. In a soup pot, combine beans with water and bay leaf. Bring to a boil and simmer partially covered for 1 1/2 hours, or until tender. In a skillet, sauté onion and celery in oil, and add to beans. If necessary, add water or stock to bring soup volume up to 6 cups. Add salt, vinegar and chard. Cook until chard is tender but still bright green, about 5 minutes.

Remove bay leaf. Serve at once.

BLACK BEAN SOUP

1 cup dried black beans
6 cups water or vegetable stock
1 onion, chopped
2 large cloves garlic, crushed
2 Tbsp. oil
2 stalks celery, coarsely chopped with leaves
1 potato, coarsely chopped
1 large carrot, coarsely chopped
2 bay leaves
1 tsp. oregano
1/4 tsp. savory
1 tsp. salt or to taste
1/8 tsp. pepper
1/4 cup fresh lemon juice

Wash beans, and place in a large saucepan with water. Cover loosely, bring to a boil and simmer for 1 1/2 hours, or until beans are not quite tender. As beans cook, add enough water or stock to yield 6 cups soup before other ingredients are added.

Meanwhile, in a skillet sauté onion and garlic in oil until soft. Add celery, potato and carrot, and heat for several minutes, stirring constantly. Add vegetables to beans. Stir in spices, salt and pepper. Bring soup to a boil, lower heat to simmer, and cook 1 hour, or until beans and vegetables are tender. Remove bay leaves. Blend soup in batches in a blender or food processor. Return to pot; add lemon juice.

COCONUT CURRY SOUP

1/4 pound rice pasta
2 tsp. cooking oil
3 cups coconut milk (canned)
2 cups vegetable broth
1 stalk lemon grass, cut into 1-inch lengths (no leaves)
4 thin slices fresh ginger
3 Tbsp. tamari
1 to 2 Tbsp. curry powder
2 tsp. grated or finely minced lime peel
2 Tbsp. lime juice
4 hot red chilies, seeded and slivered, or 2 tsp.
Chinese chili sauce or 2 tsp. hot sauce
4 oz. tofu
1 Tbsp. oriental sesame oil
8 button mushrooms
Salt to taste
Sprigs of cilantro (fresh coriander), for garnish

Bring 5 quarts of water to a rapid boil. Add the noodles and cook until just tender in the center, about 5 minutes. Immediately drain, rinse with cold water, and drain again. Mix in the cooking oil and set aside.

In a 3 quart saucepan, combine the coconut milk, broth, lemon grass, ginger, tamari, curry powder, lime peel and juice, and chilies or chili sauce. Set aside.

Cut the tofu into 1/4-inch square bite-size pieces, then mix with the sesame oil. Thinly slice the mushrooms. Set aside.
Bring the above mix to a simmer, and cook over low heat for 20 minutes. Add the tofu, and stir gently with a spoon to separate the pieces. Then add the mushrooms, noodles and salt. Serve at once.

COLD AVOCADO TOMATO MINT SOUP

1½ cups seeded and chopped tomatoes, about 1 lb.
1 cup chopped cucumber
1 ripe avocado
½ papaya, not overly ripe
1 green onion, minced
¼ cup chopped fresh mint
3 Tbsp. chopped fresh basil
3 cloves garlic, minced
3 Tbsp. lime juice
1 Tbsp. wheat free/gluten free tamari
1 tsp. Chinese chili sauce or hot sauce
¼ tsp. salt
4 cups vegetable broth

In a 6-cup bowl, add the tomatoes and cucumber. Pit the avocado, scoop out the flesh, and cut into bite-size pieces. Peel and seed the papaya, then cut into bite-size pieces. Add the avocado, papaya, green onion, mint, basil, garlic, lime juice, tamari, chili sauce or hot sauce and salt to the bowl. Stir in the broth, then refrigerate until thoroughly chilled. (This can be made a day in advance of serving).

To serve, taste the soup, and adjust the flavors of chili, lime, and salt. Ladle the soup into bowls, and top each bowl with vegetarian sour cream (see other recipe) Serve at once.

SIMPLE BLACK BEAN SOUP

1 pound black beans

2 bay leaves

1 small can tomato paste

1 large onion, diced

Salt, pepper and oregano to taste

2 Tbsp. water or oil

Bring 2 quarts of water to boil. Add beans, and boil for about 45 minutes. Drain. Sauté onion in about 2 Tbsp. oil or water in the same pan. When cooked, add the beans, seasonings, tomato paste and bay leaves, and mix carefully. Add 1 1/2 quarts of water; boil gently over low heat for about 45 minutes or until all tender.

COUNTRY BEAN SOUP

1 pound white beans or 2 cans cannellini beans (white or great northern beans)

½ cup chopped onion

1 cup tomato soup

2 tsp. minced parsley

1 cup diced celery

½ cup diced potatoes

Salt and pepper to taste

Soak beans overnight. Drain. Add fresh water, enough to cover the beans, and cook slowly, about 2 hours. Be sure never to let the water get below the level of the beans If you are using the pre-cooked canned beans; just add enough water to cover the beans. Put in onion, celery, potatoes, tomato sauce, parsley, salt and pepper. Simmer until vegetables are done; keep the water level above the level of the mixture.

Pour It On!

Salads,

Salad Dressings

and Gravies

Note: each salad dressing recipe makes enough for one large head of lettuce with toppings such as peppers, onions, etc.

PEACH SALAD DRESSING

1 peach, peeled, pit removed

2 Tbsp. lemon juice

1/4 cup safflower or olive oil

2 Tbsp. rice vinegar

Dash of freshly ground pepper

1/2 tsp. rice syrup or apple or grape juice concentrate (optional). Puree peach with lemon juice in food processor. Add remaining ingredients, and process until smooth.

TOFU SALAD

1 pound tofu, cut in finger-size pieces

1 stalk celery, diced

2 scallions, chopped

1 large white radish, chopped

Handful of parsley

1 very ripe tomato, chopped

1 Tbsp. gluten free tamari

1 tsp. oil

Pepper and salt to taste

Lettuce leaves

Arrange pieces of tofu around perimeter of plate leaving empty circle in the middle. Sprinkle with celery, scallions, radish and parsley. Put tomato in center. Drizzle all over with tamari and oil. Season. Serve on lettuce.

HINT: This salad tastes better if it sits a while before serving.

LIME DRESSING

¼ cup fresh lime juice

1 tsp. rice syrup

2 tsp. grated organic lime zest

1 tsp. minced garlic

½ cup olive oil

salt and pepper

Whisk all ingredients together until thick. Best if used at room temperature.

GINGER SALAD DRESSING

1½ cups vegetable oil

½ cup vinegar

2 Tbsp. lemon juice

dash salt

1 small minced onion

½ cup water

¼ cup wheat free/gluten free tamari

1 Tbsp. catsup

2 Tbsp. grated ginger root

Mix ingredients together and serve.

TAHINI-MISO DRESSING

1/3 cup sesame tahini

3 Tbsp. lemon juice

1 Tbsp. gluten free tamari

1 Tbsp. rice syrup

1/4 cup white miso paste

1/2 tsp. garlic powder

1/2 cup water

Handful chopped onion

Blend ingredients together.

EGGPLANT SALAD

1 eggplant

3 medium onions

3 carrots

8 tomatoes

1 tsp. garlic powder

Salt and pepper to taste

1 tsp. paprika

Oil to fry

Peel eggplant, cut in half and let drain for about **1/2** hour, then slice in bite-size pieces. Chop the onions, and sauté until translucent; add the eggplant and onions until just brown. (Add more oil if necessary). Peel tomatoes by dropping them in hot water for about 30 seconds. After peeling the tomatoes, grate them, and add them together with the grated carrots to the eggplant and onion mixture. Season with salt, pepper, garlic powder and paprika; cook on slow fire for about 30 minutes.

Best eaten when cold as an appetizer.

MUSHROOM SAGE GRAVY

4 cups mushrooms, sliced (any kind of mushrooms will do)

1/2 cup apple juice

1 tsp. sage

1 cup rice milk or non-dairy milk

2 Tbsp. cornstarch or arrowroot

Sauté mushrooms, apple juice and sage over low heat for approximately 20 minutes. Sprinkle in cornstarch while stirring. (This should make a thick paste). Slowly add milk. Stir to avoid lumps.

This is good over brown rice, baked potatoes or even wheat free/gluten free pasta.

MUSHROOM-ONION GRAVY

3 Tbsp. olive oil
1 medium onion, diced
1 clove garlic, minced
1 cup sliced mushrooms
1 Tbsp. nutritional yeast
2 Tbsp. rice flour
2 Tbsp. powdered vegetable broth or wheat free/gluten free tamari
1 1/2 cups water or vegetable broth

Sauté vegetables in oil for 3-4 minutes. Stir in flour, yeast and vegetable powder or tamari. Add water or broth, slowly, stirring with a whisk until smooth.

"TUNA FISH" SALAD

1 cup carrots, finely grated (approximately 3-4 carrots)
3 celery stalks, minced
3 Tbsp. lemon juice
1/2 Tbsp. wheat free tamari
1/2 Tbsp. kelp or nori seaweed seasoning (optional, but it helps give it the fish taste if that is what you like)
1/2 cup green onions, chopped

Finely grate the carrots in a food processor, then transfer to a mixing bowl. Add the other ingredients, mix well and refrigerate. Great on sandwiches or any place you use regular tuna salad. Serve in celery ribs, on bell pepper wedges or on top of a salad.

CUCUMBER SALAD

3 cucumbers, sliced

½ cup vinegar

1 small onion, minced

Pepper to taste

Mix ingredients together. This can be served immediately; however, it tastes better if allowed to sit in the refrigerator for a day or two. Store in a jar.

ANOTHER "TUNA" SALAD

1 cup garbanzo beans (canned or precooked)

1 stalk celery, chopped

½ small onion, minced finely

Mayonnaise (see other recipe or use commercial vegan mayonnaise)

Salt and pepper to taste

Mash the garbanzo beans (chickpeas). Add remaining ingredients, and mix well. Spread on bread as a sandwich, or serve on lettuce.

TOMATO BASIL SALAD

6 large tomatoes, cubed

1 tsp. chopped fresh basil

3 Tbsp. lemon juice (optional)

1 small onion, finely chopped

2 cloves garlic, crushed (optional)

Black pepper to taste

Mix together. Serve cold. This may seem real simple, but it is the most incredible way I have found to eat tomatoes. It goes well with a few slices of lightly toasted wheat free/gluten free bread.

AVOCADO - CASHEW DRESSING

Blend until smooth:

1/2 cups raw cashews

1 1/2 cups hot water

Add and continue to blend

2 avocados

2 tsp. lemon juice

Cool before serving

For a dip, add 1/2 medium size onion to the first ingredients.

AVOCADO DRESSING

1/2 cup orange juice or apple juice

1 Tbsp. lemon juice

1/4 tsp. salt

1 avocado, mashed

Blend and serve.

CUCUMBER DRESSING

Blend until smooth:

3/4 cup raw cashews

3/4 cup hot water

1/2 cucumber (peeled if not organic)

4 green onions

Cool.

Add before using:

1/4 cup minced parsley (optional)

1/4 cup diced radishes (optional)

1 tsp. salt and herbs (your choices)

Fresh or dried cilantro, rosemary and thyme

ANOTHER FRENCH DRESSING

1/2 cup lemon juice

1/2 tsp. salt

1/4 cup raw cashews

1/2 tsp. paprika

1/3 cup water

Garlic, onion and dill as desired

Blend and serve.

ITALIAN DRESSING

1/3 cup lemon juice

3 cups pineapple juice

1 tsp. celery seed

1 tsp. crushed dried basil

1 tsp. onion powder

Blend and serve.

MEXICAN FRUIT SALAD

2 cups fresh pineapple

1 small jicama

1 large mango (not too soft)

1 tsp. jalapeno pepper, chopped

2 Tbsp. packed cilantro leaves, chopped

1 lime, juiced

1 tsp. poppy seeds

Chop the pineapple, jicama and mango; put them into a bowl.

Put the jalapeno chunks through a garlic press, and press their juice onto the fruit; discard the fibers inside the press.

Chop the cilantro leaves, and add to the other spices.

Chill.

PAPAYA KIWI SALAD

1 small papaya

1 kiwi

1/4 cup raisins

1 lime, cut in half (juice one half, slice thinly the other half)

Peel and slice the papaya into small spears; peel and quarter the kiwis. Arrange the papaya and kiwi on a beautiful platter, and sprinkle the raisins and lime juice. Garnish with lime slices.

LEMON-TARRAGON SALAD DRESSING

2 Tbsp. finely chopped fresh tarragon

1 Tbsp. fresh lemon juice

1/3 cup olive oil

Salt and freshly ground pepper

In a large bowl, combine the tarragon and lemon juice. Gradually whisk in the oil, and season with salt and pepper.

BLACK BEAN SALAD

2 large onions

6 large carrots, diced

1 cup sliced napa cabbage

2 tsp. onion salt

2 cloves crushed garlic

1½ tsp. chili powder

¼ tsp. cayenne pepper (optional)

3 tsp. fresh dill, cut very fine

1 tsp. fresh basil, cut very fine

½ tsp. black pepper

1 bay leaf (optional)

9 large scallions cut in 1/2-inch pieces

2 15 oz. cans black beans (do not drain)

2 cups chopped spinach

5 plum tomatoes, diced

2 Tbsp. fresh lemon juice

Slice onions into 1-inch strips. Spray or lightly coat a large pot with olive oil, and place over medium heat. Sauté onions until translucent, about 2 minutes. Add carrots, cabbage and spices. Sauté 5 to 10 minutes, until carrots soften. Add scallions and sauté another 10 minutes, until vegetables are slightly undercooked. Stir in black beans, including liquid, then add spinach. Cook another 5 minutes, then add tomatoes. Cook until tomatoes are heated through, then add lemon juice just before serving.

CAESAR SALAD

Servings: Makes about 8 side dish servings of salad.

DRESSING:

1 Tbsp. minced garlic

2 tsp. Dijon mustard

2 tsp. umeboshi plum paste *OR* 2 more tsp. Dijon mustard

3 Tbsp. balsamic vinegar

3 Tbsp. lemon juice

1 Tbsp. light miso

½ 10½-oz. package soft silken tofu

1⅓ cup extra-virgin olive oil

2 heads Romaine lettuce, washed, dried and

Chilled dulse powder (a dried seaweed) to taste

Dressing: Combine all dressing ingredients except oils in bowl, blender or food processor; whisk or blend until creamy. In a thin stream, add oils; blend until fully mixed together.

To Serve: Tear lettuce into bite-sized pieces, toss with dressing. Add dulse powder to taste.

BEET SALAD WITH SCALLIONS

1 pound beets

4 scallions, thinly sliced

¼ cup lemon juice

2 Tbsp. olive oil

¼ cup minced fresh mint

salt and pepper to taste

4 lettuce leaves

Preheat oven to 375°. Trim greens from beets; place beets on cookie sheet. Roast until tender when pricked with a fork, 45 to 60 minutes.

Peel and quarter beets; shred in food processor, and transfer to a serving bowl. Add remaining ingredients and toss. Chill, and serve on top of lettuce leaves.

DR. JOE'S SIGNATURE SALAD

1 ripe avocado, peeled

2 ripe medium tomatoes

2 ripe mangos

Cut all ingredients into ¼-inch cubes. Hint: cut avocado in half, remove the pit, then cut 2 halves in half again, and just peel back the skin and cut into ½ inch cubes.

Peel the mangos with a potato peeler or knife; cut the flesh away from the pit, then cube. (Continued on next page.)

THE DRESSING
for Dr. Joe's Signature Salad

Juice of 2 limes

3 Tbsp. thinly sliced fresh basil

2 Tbsp. wheat free tamari

2 Tbsp. rice syrup

1/4 tsp. Chinese chili sauce or hot sauce

Mix dressing with fruits and serve!

FRENCH DRESSING

Whiz the following in a blender until smooth:

1 cup tomato puree

2 Tbsp. rice syrup or apple or grape juice concentrate

1/2 cup lemon juice

1 clove garlic

Then stir in the following:

2 tsp. Italian seasoning or oregano

1 tsp. dill weed

1 tsp. dried salt

Chill and Serve. Keep refrigerated. Use within 7 to 8 days.

CREAMY ITALIAN DRESSING

Mix together the following in a saucepan:

1 cup cold water

⅔ cup lemon juice

2 tsp. garlic powder

4 tsp. Italian seasoning or oregano

2 tsp. onion powder

1 tsp. salt

1 tsp. rice syrup or apple or grape juice concentrate

2 tsp. cornstarch

Then bring the above to a boil stirring constantly. Remove from heat, and chill thoroughly. Keep refrigerated. Use within 7 to 8 days.

MIXED MUSHROOM SALAD

SALAD

1 pound mixed mushrooms (button, shiitake, enoki, oyster)
½ pound jicama
1 sweet red pepper
3 cups bean sprouts
6 Tbsp. chopped fresh parsley

DRESSING

2 Tbsp. very thinly sliced fresh ginger
1 clove garlic
¼ cup chopped green onions
5 Tbsp. white wine vinegar
¼ cup mild olive oil
3 Tbsp. oriental sesame oil
2 Tbsp. tamari
2 Tbsp. apple juice
¼ tsp. freshly ground black pepper

Cut the button mushrooms into thin slices. Discard the stems from the shiitake mushrooms, and cut the caps into eighths. Cut the dirty ends off the enoki mushrooms, and separate the long stems. Cut the oyster mushrooms into quarters or eighths.

Peel the jicama. Cut into bite-size rectangles about 1/4-inch thick. Cut the pepper into the same size pieces. Set aside the jicama, pepper, sprouts and parsley.

Place the ginger and garlic in a food processor and finely mince. Add the remaining dressing ingredients, and blend for 30 seconds.

About 30 minutes before serving, toss the mushrooms in the dressing. Just before serving, stir in the jicama, pepper, sprouts and parsley. Serve at once.

COLD BEAN SALAD

2 cups cooked pinto beans

2 cups cooked garbanzo beans

2 cups cooked kidney beans

2 stalks celery, diced

1 green pepper, diced

1 small onion, diced

1 Tbsp. molasses or rice syrup

3 Tbsp. nutritional yeast

½ tsp. sea salt

½ tsp. garlic powder

¼ tsp. paprika

¼ tsp. oregano

¼ tsp. basil

⅛ tsp. red pepper

2 cloves garlic, minced

½ cup oil

3 Tbsp. wheat free/gluten free tamari

2 Tbsp. apple cider vinegar

Combine beans, celery, green pepper and onion in a large bowl. Blend remaining ingredients in a blender or food processor on high for one minute. Add to bean/vegetable mixture, and stir well. Chill for 2 hours to marinate.

SHIITAKE MUSHROOM GRAVY

2 Tbsp. olive oil

½ cup brown rice flour

¼ pound fresh shiitake mushrooms, sliced

2 Tbsp. fresh marjoram or thyme

1 quart vegetable stock

2 Tbsp. tamari

1 tsp. apple cider vinegar

Sea salt and freshly ground black pepper

Heat oil in a 2-quart saucepan. Add rice flour, and stir with a wooden spoon until the mixture becomes the consistency of wet sand. Add mushrooms, and cook 5 minutes more.

Pour in stock and tamari. Bring to a slow boil, and cook 20 to 30 minutes until thickened. Adjust seasoning with apple cider vinegar, sea salt and black pepper.

SIMPLE ITALIAN DRESSING

Equal parts Balsamic vinegar and good quality olive oil. Generous amount of garlic powder. Salt and pepper to taste. Mix all together.

Pour on salad. This is the salad dressing that made my mom famous. It is great over bitter greens like endive or radish tops.

ASPARAGUS ROLL-UPS

Servings: Makes 16 roll-ups

Use soft lettuces such as butter or red oak for this appetizer or salad:

1 cup vegetarian mayonnaise (can be purchased in
health food section of your grocery store)

1 Tbsp. chopped sun-dried tomatoes in oil

3 scallions, finely chopped (white and green parts)

16 lettuce leaves, washed and dried

32 large asparagus spears, lightly cooked and drained

16 sprigs fresh dill weed

Steamed scallion strips (optional)

Edible flowers (optional)*

In a small bowl, mix mayonnaise, sun-dried tomatoes and chopped scallions. With a tsp., spread a little mixture inside each lettuce leaf. Top with 2 asparagus spears. Add 1 sprig dill weed and 1 edible flower if desired. Roll to form a "bouquet"; tie with scallion strips. Place on a serving platter. Repeat until all ingredients are used. Chill until ready to serve.

*Edible flowers can be purchased at most farmers markets or gourmet food stores. This is a nice touch but not necessary.

BASIL DRESSING

2 Tbsp. dry onion

1 cup hot water

½ cup raw cashews

½ tsp. salt

1 tsp. fresh basil, finely chopped

2 Tbsp. lemon juice

10 olives

Blend.

EGGLESS EGG SALAD

1 pound firm tofu, drained

1½ tsp. apple cider vinegar

3 tsp. prepared yellow mustard

½ tsp. turmeric

2 Tbsp. diced celery & onion

1 tsp. parsley, chopped

½ tsp. white pepper

dash paprika

Crumble tofu in a bowl, and set aside. In a separate bowl, combine next four ingredients, mix well and pour over tofu. Add remaining ingredients, mix well; refrigerate 30 minutes. Great on top of lettuce or in a sandwich.

POTATO SALAD

6 cooked cubed potatoes

1 small onion, thinly sliced

1 medium cucumber, thinly sliced

Dressing:

1 cup water

1 Tbsp. poultry seasoning

1 Tbsp. dill seed

½ cup cashews

1 Tbsp. lemon juice

Sea salt as needed

Blend dressing ingredients; mix lightly with potato mixture and chill for several hours.

TOFU MAYONNAISE

1 cup (packed) mashed firm tofu

1 small clove garlic

1 tsp. prepared mustard (brown or Dijon taste best)

2 tsp. cider vinegar

¼ to ½ tsp. salt

¼ cup olive oil (optional)

2 tsp. lemon juice

Place ingredients in a food processor fitted with the steel blade or in a blender. Process until very creamy and smooth. Place in sealed container in refrigerator, and it will keep for several weeks. You can vary the flavor by adding fresh minced herbs, garlic, lemon peel or pepper.

OTHER SPREADS

Puree ½ cup tofu mayonnaise with the following ingredients to create several new and wonderful spreads.

Cilantro-lime	½ cup loosely packed cilantro leaves and 2 tsp. lime juice
Sun-dried tomato	4 sun-dried tomatoes in oil
Kalamata olive	¼ cup Kalamata olives
Basil-lemon	⅓ cup loosely packed basil leaves and 1 Tbsp. lemon juice
Sesame-ginger	½ tsp. sesame oil and 1½ Tbsp. grated fresh ginger
Wasabi	1½ tsp. Wasabi paste
Rice syrup-Dijon	1 Tbsp. rice syrup and 1 Tbsp. Dijon mustard
Provencal	2 Tbsp. rinsed, drained capers and ½ tsp. fresh thyme
Garlic	1 clove garlic, crushed in a press
Horseradish	1 Tbsp. prepared horseradish

VEGETABLE BUTTER

¾ cup cold water

4 Tbsp. fine yellow cornmeal or corn flour

¾ cup reduced-fat, extra-firm silken or medium-firm

regular tofu, well drained

¼ cup water

¾ tsp. salt

Mix the cold water and cornmeal or flour together in a small, heavy saucepan. Cook over medium-heat, stirring constantly until the mixture is quite thick. Cover, and cook over low heat for 5 minutes more.

Scrape into a blender with a spatula, and add the remaining ingredients.

Blend until very smooth. Pour into a tightly covered, wide mouth container, and refrigerate. This firms up nicely when chilled and melts well on hot food.

*This lasts for about 5 days.

GREEN BEAN & MUSHROOM SALAD

¼ cup red vinegar

1 tsp. vegetable oil

1 Tbsp. chopped parsley

1 cup mushrooms, button or other

3 cups green beans (fresh or frozen)

pepper and garlic powder to taste

Steam green beans, if fresh, until tender crisp. Place in a bowl with ice water to keep them green. When cool, or if using thawed frozen, add mushrooms sliced, vinegar, oil and chopped parsley. Combine all ingredients. Mix well, and cover. Refrigerate for at least 1 hour.

GREEN ONION DRESSING

4 oz. tofu, drained

5 whole green onions

2 Tbsp. red vinegar

2 Tbsp. lemon juice (fresh)

¼ tsp. black pepper

Combine ingredients in a blender. Blend until smooth. Serve over lettuce or any vegetables or as a dip.

GREEN GODDESS DRESSING

4 oz. tofu, pressed under a paper towel

to get most of the water out

1/4 cup rice vinegar

2 stalks celery (washed)

2 raw spinach leaves (washed)

8 large sprigs fresh parsley

1/8 tsp. each tarragon & black pepper

1 clove garlic

1/4 cup lemon juice

Combine in blender. Blend until smooth. Serve over your favorite raw vegetables as you would any salad dressing or as a dip.

HAZELNUT VINEGARETTE DRESSING

3 Tbsp. Dijon mustard

3 Tbsp. shallot, chopped

1 tsp. garlic, chopped

1 tsp. salt

½ tsp. white pepper

6 oz. tarragon vinegar

20 oz. hazelnut oil

12 oz. olive oil

1 Tbsp. tarragon, chopped

1 Tbsp. parsley, chopped

1 tsp. hot sauce

Mix the first 6 ingredients in a large bowl. Slowly add the oils to the mixture in a steady manner while whipping. This can be done in a blender or food processor, providing the unit has a bowl large enough to handle the volume. After the oils have been added, add the tarragon, parsley and hot sauce. Place in a sealed container, and refrigerate. This makes a lot of dressing so you can ½ or even ¼ the recipe to try it out the first time, but most people like it enough to make it all.

Delicious Dips & Splendid Spreads

HUMMUS (GARBANZO BEAN SPREAD)

2 cups garbanzo paste (cook your own beans as described below or use canned beans)
½ cup sesame seeds ground in a food processor or blender (or use pre-made tahini, which is sesame seed butter)
Juice of 1 lemon
½ tsp. cumin, ground
1 to 2 tsp. paprika
2 cloves garlic, mashed
¼ cup fresh cilantro, minced (optional)
½ Olive oil
1 tsp air dried sea salt

Soak garbanzo beans overnight in enough water to cover them, or bring the beans to a boil for one minute, also in enough water to cover them.

Cover the beans, and set them aside for one or more hours. Drain the beans, and cover them again with fresh water. Cook over medium heat for 2½ hours or until tender. In food processor with the steel "S" blade or blender, process until the beans are smooth. Grind the sesame seeds in a blender or food processor until they become paste. Add the seeds to the beans, and process until the spread is well combined. Add the remaining ingredients. Mix thoroughly.

Try this: Hummus is great on bread with lettuce, tomato, sprouts, celery, carrot dip or just plain.

VEGGIE SOUR CREAM

1 10.5 oz. package firm silken tofu, drained

3 Tbsp. vegetable oil

1 tsp. brown rice syrup

Juice of 1 lemon

½ tsp. salt, or to taste

Blend all ingredients until very smooth in a blender or food processor.

GUACAMOLE

2 medium avocados, mashed

2 tsp. jalapenos, minced

½ cup tomato, chopped fine, or ½ c. salsa

1 Tbsp. lime juice

1 tsp. garlic, minced

1 Tbsp. red onion, minced

2 Tbsp. cilantro, minced

Cracked pepper and sea salt to taste

Garnish: 1 Tbsp. green onion, minced

Mash avocados with a fork in a small bowl. Stir in the remaining ingredients. To prevent avocados from discoloring, place the avocado pit on top before storing or serve immediately.

Try this: Add 2 Tbsp. nutritional yeast to the above for a great and healthy new taste.

TOFU SPINACH DIP

½ pound tofu

2 Tbsp. mustard or mayonnaise

10 oz. box frozen spinach or fresh cooked

1 large onion, chopped

2 cloves garlic minced

2 Tbsp. oil

dash pepper and tamari to taste

Sauté onions and garlic in oil. Pour into blender, add remaining ingredients and blend well. Serve with crackers or raw vegetables.

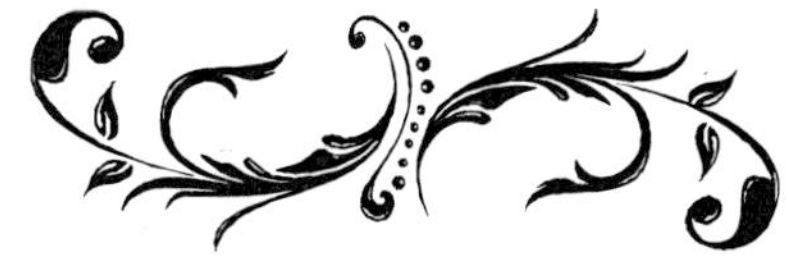

Blissful Beverages

Milks and Creams and Other Drinks

NUT MILK OR NUT CREAM

2 cups raw cashews, walnuts or almonds

4 cups hot water

2 Tbsp. rice syrup or 8 pitted dates

½ Tbsp. vanilla

Dash of salt

Whip in a blender or food processor until liquid, and cool before serving.

For milk, use 5 cups water.

"CHOCOLATE" MILK

1 cup nut milk

Add:

2 Tbsp. maple syrup

1 tsp. carob powder

½ tsp. vanilla

Strain, chill or serve warm.

For smoothies:

Blend the "chocolate" milk or any nut milk with frozen bananas or frozen peaches for a wonderful milkshake.

QUICK ALMOND MILK

½ cup almonds

3 cups distilled water

For creamy white nut milk, blanch almonds by pouring very hot (almost boiling) water over them to loosen skins.

Remove skins by pinching each almond between your thumb and index finger.

Place almonds in one bowl and skins in another.

Blend blanched almonds with distilled water, using highest blender speed for three minutes. For a real wild treat, add ¼ tsp. vanilla and/or 1 tsp. rice syrup.

Delightful!

If you choose not to blanch almonds, use them whole or grind them in a nut-and-seed grinder or food mill, then blend almonds (or almond meal) on high speed with water.

Strain, and serve cold, or serve hot on a cold night with added cinnamon or nutmeg.

RICE MILK

⅓ cups hot cooked rice

⅓ cup cashew meal (cashews ground into a meal, but not ground enough to be cashew butter)

1 tsp. vanilla

½ tsp. salt

2 Tbsp. rice syrup or 4 pitted dates

3 cups hot water

Place in a blender, and blend until smooth. Chill, and serve anywhere you would use regular milk.

OATMEAL MILK

2 cups cooked gluten free oatmeal

4 cups water

½ tsp. salt

1 ripe banana

1 tsp. vanilla

2 Tbsp. rice syrup or 4 pitted dates

Place in a blender, and blend until smooth. Chill and use anywhere you would use regular milk.

Note: Many individuals, who have wheat allergies, also have oatmeal allergies, so if you do - do not use this milk. The protein in oatmeal is similar in structure to the protein in oatmeal, even with certified gluten free oats; some individuals may not be able to tolerate oats.

SESAME MILK

1 cup sesame seeds

¼ tsp. salt

2 cups water

¼ cup rice syrup or 6 pitted dates

Bring sesame seeds and water to a boil, and simmer 10 minutes. Place in a blender, add the other ingredients and blend until smooth. Chill, and use anywhere you would use regular milk.

HOMEMADE SODA

8 oz. seltzer (salt free)

2 Tbsp. frozen juice concentrate

(orange, grape, lemon, grapefruit, apple, etc.)

Pour chilled seltzer into a glass. Add frozen juice concentrate. Stir well and serve.

Try this: Add ½ cup juice instead of frozen concentrate to ½ cup of seltzer. Stir, and serve. Add a twist of lemon or lime for added fun.

HOT APPLE CIDER

½ gallon apple cider

1 lemon, sliced thinly

1 or 2 tsp. cinnamon

¼ tsp. nutmeg

Heat above ingredients in a large pot over a medium heat, stirring occasionally, until heated through.

SWEET HOT OR ICED TEA

Use 1 cup of your favorite hot non-citrus juice (such as apple or grape) instead of water with 1 tea bag when making your favorite naturally caffeine-free herbal tea. This makes it naturally sweet. For iced tea, just ice down the above for a great summer drink.

How Sweet It Is!

Fruit Meals, Sweets & Snacks

BANANA DATE SMOOTHIE

2-4 dried dates, pitted

1 cup fresh fruit juice

2 frozen bananas (peel and cut fresh bananas in half and place in plastic bag or plastic container to freeze)

Use freshly-made apple, grape or pear juice as a base or commercially made juice if fresh is not available. Place juice in blender; pit dates; add pitted dates to juice; blend at high speed. (Dried apples may also be used and added at this time.)

Add frozen bananas, one-half banana at a time, through opening in blender lid while blender is running on high speed. (A relatively small amount of fresh ripe bananas may also be used if desired.)

This creamy-smooth drink is a meal in itself. Lip-Smackin' good!

CAROB SUNDAE OR BANANA SPLIT

½ cup freshly-made fruit juice

2-4 dates, preferably soft ones, pitted

3 Tbsp. carob powder, preferably unroasted

Banana Ice Cream, Strawberry-Banana Ice Cream, and/or Ban-Apple Ice Cream

Pour juice into blender, pit and add several (soft) dates and liquefy them in liquid until well blended. Carefully add carob powder, and blend in, stopping blender to stir or add more carob powder or liquid as needed and then replacing blender lid and blending again. Carob syrup should be medium-thick (not watery) and smooth. Use a narrow plastic spatula to get most of the syrup into a bowl or other container. (You can make a surplus and store it in your refrigerator. If you do this, you may want to pour carob syrup into a storage container with a tight fitting lid.)

Make ice cream, and scoop carob syrup on top. You may wish to sprinkle some raisins on top.

This makes a smashingly wholesome meal!

Serve over bananas to make a Banana Split!

PINEAPPLE SHERBET

½ cup pineapple, fresh and removed from husk

½ cup fresh strawberries, washed, de-stemmed and sliced

Blend pineapple until smooth in a blender, and pour into a freezer container.

Freeze until semi-hard and then stir well, and fold in sliced strawberries.

Freeze overnight.

*Note many people have allergic reactions to strawberries and/or pineapple. If you itch or if your lips, tongue or skin break out after tasting this, you should avoid strawberries and pineapple.

PLUM PUDDING

2 plums

1 banana, peeled and frozen

Wash and halve fresh plums; remove pits; place plums in blender, and liquefy on high speed.

With blender still running on high speed, add frozen peeled bananas through opening in blender lid, a half banana at a time, until mixture becomes thick, stopping blender and stirring when necessary.

You may use all or partly fresh bananas, but frozen bananas make the pudding thicker and colder.

Serve immediately - plain or with sliced bananas or other fresh fruit on top or mixed in.

NECTARINE PUDDING

2 fresh nectarines

Wash nectarines; remove pits; place fruit in blender, and liquefy on high speed until creamy and smooth.

Serve this pudding plain or with a few blueberries, soaked raisins (or other cut-up soaked dried fruit), sliced banana or any other kind of diced fresh fruit on top or mixed in. (Peaches, apricots, plums, grapes, and berries combine best with this pudding.)

BANANA-PEACH PUDDING

1 ripe banana

1 fresh peach

Peel very ripe banana(s) and break in half.

Place bananas in blender, and liquefy on high speed.

Wash peach; remove pit; add to blended banana, and blend again on high speed until liquefied.

Serve with or without diced fresh and/or soaked dried fruit on top or mixed in.

This pudding is delectable and simple to prepare.

*Note: If you wish, you may use peeled and frozen bananas instead of or in addition to fresh bananas to make this pudding thicker and colder. If you use frozen bananas, liquefy peaches (and/or fresh bananas) first, then add frozen bananas through opening in blender lid while blender is running.

BANANA SOUP

6-10 bananas

1½ cup unsweetened coconut (shredded or grated)

1½ cup raisins

Liquefy bananas on highest blender speed, and pour into a saucepan.

Stir in shredded or grated coconut. While heating the mixture a bit, add and stir in raisins.

Heat only until warm.

Slice another banana on top if desired.

PAPAYA SOUP

1 cup ripe papaya, cubed

1 frozen ripe banana

¼ cup of your favorite fruit juice

Peel and freeze ripe banana in a plastic bag.

Cut papaya in half, and scoop out the seeds with a spoon. Then scoop out the flesh from skins, and place into a blender.

Next, put frozen bananas in a food processor with an "S" shaped blade; add the juice, and whip until creamy. Put the creamy banana into the blender, and blend just enough to mostly mix the banana with the papaya, stopping the blender and stirring with a spoon if necessary.

Serve immediately.

Note: A blender can be used instead of a food processor if you are in a pinch.

ALL FRUIT PIE CRUST

Servings: 2 crusts

½ cup dehydrated pineapple

½ cup dehydrated papaya

1 cup raisins

3 cups dehydrated bananas

or

2 cups almonds, finely chopped in a food processor

In a food processor (using the "S" blade) combine all ingredients. Allow processor to run until all of the ingredients are pulverized. The mixture should become one mass and begin to move in slow circles around the inside of the food processor. This takes a few minutes so do not get impatient. Press it into a pie pan to an even thickness of ¼" to ⅜". Greasing the pan with a little vegetable oil before placing in the crust will help prevent it from sticking. You may now fill it with one of the filling recipes or, as you become more experienced, make your own pie filling. Once the pie is complete, refrigerate overnight, and serve by slicing the pie with a very sharp knife. Be careful, these pies can be habit forming and you may never want to eat another type of pie again.

STRAWBERRY PIE FILLING

Servings: 1 pie

1½ pints fresh strawberries

2 bananas

3 kiwis

¼ pineapple

Cut one banana, 3 kiwis, ½ pint strawberries and ¼ pineapple into small slices. Line the bottom of a pie crust with the fruit slices laid flat. Next combine 1 pint of strawberries and 1 banana in a food processor using the "S" blade. Process the fruit until pureed.

*Note: Many people are allergic to strawberries, and/or pineapple. If your lips or tongue break out after eating these fruits, simply avoid them.

APPLE PIE FILLING

Makes filling for 1 pie

5 medium sized golden delicious or red apples

1¼ tsp. apple pie spice or allspice

3 Tbsp. lemon juice or lime juice

1 cup dried pineapple, raisin or papaya

½ cup banana chips (optional)

Remove the skin and core from four apples. Cut 4 apples into chunks and place in a food processor with the "S" blade. Add apple pie spice, lemon juice and pineapples, raisins or papaya. Process until smooth. Take the remaining apple, and cut into thin slices to be placed on the bottom of the pie. Pour mixture over sliced apples into the pie crust. Top with crushed banana chips, raisins or papaya. Refrigerate until firm, at least 2 hours.

Serve.

SWEET POTATO PIE FILLING

Makes filling for 1 pie

4 cups finely shredded sweet potatoes

½ cup hot water

1 tsp. pumpkin pie spice

2 tsp. vanilla extract

2 tsp. rice syrup

2 tsp. lemon juice

Blend all ingredients in a blender or food processor until mixture is smooth (about 3 minutes). Filling should not have a gritty texture when tasted. Apply filling to all fruit pie crust and smooth out with a spatula processor.

Cover with plastic wrap, and refrigerate until ready to serve.

POP'S POPS (invented by my father)

2 ripe bananas peeled, cut up and frozen

1 cup of your favorite fruit juice
  (apple, peach, cherry, etc.)

Ice pop molds or very small paper cups

With popsicle sticks

Whip bananas and juice in the blender until smooth, pour into molds or cups, and place one stick in each cup. Freeze overnight, and take out of cup or mold and eat.

THE FAMOUS BREAKFAST SHAKE

2 bananas, peeled, cut and frozen in a plastic bag or container

2 cups of your favorite fruit juice such as grape, apple, pear etc. or any "milk" (see "milk" recipes)

1 apple, cored

Or

2 pitted peaches

Or

2 cups cleaned grapes

Or

2 cups of your favorite berries

Or

2 diced mangos

Or

2 more bananas or whatever fresh fruit you like

Place in a food processor or blender, and whip until smooth. More juice will make it smoother, less juice will make it thicker. Peaches and berries freeze well and can be added.

This is the perfect breakfast meal and can be eaten on your way to work or school.

FROZEN NO-BAKE BIRTHDAY CAKE

1 Bunt Cake Pan
16 oz. of dried organic figs, soaked overnight in distilled water
16 oz. of dried pitted organic dates, soaked overnight in distilled water
12 oz. bag of organic almonds
2 big bunches of fully ripened bananas (organic if possible)

Soak fruit in separate bowls. The water level for soaking is about half full. Do not cover the dried fruits completely. Remove stems from soaked figs, puree figs and set aside. Puree dates put in separate bowl, chop almonds in food processor or blender and set aside in its own container. Peel and puree the bananas in a blender or food processor.

CREATING THE CAKE

Place almonds in the bottom of the Bunt cake pan; 2nd layer, pureed figs; 3rd layer almonds; 4th layer pureed bananas, almonds, dates, almond, figs or whatever order you desire. Almonds should be the first layer and end with dates or figs the last layer. Cover, and freeze overnight.

TO SERVE

Remove from the freezer, place upside down on a plate and allow to sit a few minutes until thawed enough to release from the pan. The pan can be carefully set in warm water right side up just long enough to release the cake then place it upside down, but be very careful not to get water in the cake. Place a sharp knife in hot water to warm it up and help it slice better.

Cut, and enjoy.

BANANA CREAM PUDDING OR PIE

2 ripe bananas

1 cup raw cashews

2 cups hot water

2 to 4 dates

½ tsp. salt

4 Tbsp. cornstarch or arrow root

Place cashews, 1 cup hot water, dates, vanilla, 1 banana and salt in a blender or food processor, and blend until smooth. Mix 1 cup hot water with corn starch or arrowroot, add to mixture and cool until thick. Top with the other banana, sliced or to make a pie simply pour into the all fruit pie crust, and refrigerate until cold.

RICE PUDDING

½ cup raw brown rice

2 cups apple juice

⅛ Tbsp. salt

½ cup raisins

Combine the above, and bring to a boil. Cover, and cook on low heat for 40 minutes or until rice is soft. Add:

1 cup chopped dates

1½ cup diced apples

Cook 10 minutes longer. Top with nuts, and serve plain or with cashew cream.

DATE AND COCONUT PIE

1½ cups coconut, freshly grated, for the crust

⅓ cup water (or fruit juice)

3 large bananas

⅔ cup pitted dates

⅔ cup grated coconut (for the topping)

⅓ cup pitted dates, sliced

Moisten the freshly grated coconut with a bit of water, and pat the mix into the pie plate for crust.

Chill the crust for an hour or so. Blend the bananas and the ⅔ cup pitted dates in as little water as possible. This mixture should be quite thick. Pour the pie filling into the crust. Top the pie with the ⅔ cup shredded coconut and the ⅓ cup of sliced dates. Chill for at least 2 hours, and serve.

HOME MADE ICE CREAMS

Strawberries, peaches, apricots, or any frozen fruit

Freeze the berries or fruit of choice; put them into a food processor or blender. Blend until smooth, adding enough juice to blend. Serve immediately, or freeze 1 hour to firm up your fresh fruit dessert before serving it.

BLUEBERRY ICE CREAM

½ cup tofu, soft

1½ cup frozen blueberries

2 Tbsp. rice syrup or apple or grape juice concentrate, few drops peppermint oil or extract

Blend all until smooth - great after fiery spicy foods.

PINA COLADA SORBET

2 cups pineapple chunks

1 banana

¼ cup pineapple coconut juice or orange juice

½ cup shredded coconut

Freeze the pineapple overnight.

Blend or puree the frozen pineapple with the banana and coconut, adding the juice slowly. Stop and stir until it is all pureed - put into glasses or dessert cups, and freeze for 1 hour before serving.

BANANA ICE CREAM

2 bananas

½ to ⅓ cups juice or nut milk

Peel ripe but not mushy bananas, and cut into 5 or 6 pieces. Place into a plastic bag, and freeze solid. This will take at least a day. Blend bananas in a food processor or blender with liquid. Use just enough liquid to turn bananas into puree, but not too much. We do not want a smoothie texture. Occasionally turn off the machine, and push bananas down toward the blades with a rubber spatula. Eat as is, or place in the freezer for about another ½ to one hour to make a firmer ice cream.

MAPLE WALNUT ICE CREAM

2 frozen bananas

1⅓ cup water

2 Tbsp. walnuts or pecans

⅛ tsp. vanilla

1⅛ tsp. maple syrup

1⁄16 tsp. salt

Follow the directions for banana ice cream using the ingredients above.

CAROB ICE CREAM

2 frozen bananas

1⅓ cup “chocolate” milk (see page 195)

Follow the directions for banana ice cream using the ingredients above.

GOLDEN MACAROONS

1 cup grated raw carrots, packed

½ cup water

⅓ cup rice syrup

1½ cup shredded coconut

1 cup rice flour

½ Tbsp. salt

1 tsp. vanilla

Mix all the ingredients very well. Let stand 10 minutes. Firmly pack dough into a tablespoon, then drop on an oiled cookie sheet. Bake at 325° for 30 minutes.

FRUIT CAKE

For one large or two small cakes:

1 pound coconut meal, unsweetened
(shredded may be used if meal is unavailable)
1 pound nuts (pecans, almonds or walnuts)
12 oz. soaked dried fruit (figs, raisins) and/or dried dates
(no need to soak the dates)
8-10 medium bananas
2 cups fresh fruit
(plums, peaches, apples, pears, pineapple, strawberries, etc.)

Soak dried fruit in hot water for 3 hours or in room temperature over night. Take the fruit out of the water, and liquefy soaked dried fruit (and/or dates) on highest blender speed, using soak water (and/or distilled water) as needed.

Grind nuts (and coconut, if shredded and not a meal) in a nut and seed grinder or blender.

Place nuts and coconut in a large mixing bowl; add blended fruit mixture; mix well, using your hands rather than a spoon. At this point, the mixture should be moist but hold together. Add more nuts/coconut or water if needed.

Slice fresh fruit into bite-size pieces, add to mixture and mix in with your hands.

Place mixture evenly in one large rectangular or two small square cake pans, and sprinkle coconut on top.

Place cake in freezer for several hours or overnight. When cake is just barely frozen but firm, it's ready to eat. (If the cake is frozen solid, let it partially thaw 1-3 hours or so before serving.)

APPLE PIE WITH MILLET CRUST

Servings: 1 pie

1/4 cup pumpkin seeds

1/3 cup millet, rinsed well

1/2 cup apple juice or cider

7 medium sweet apples, grated

1/8 tsp. sea salt

1/2 tsp. cinnamon

1 Tbsp. arrowroot

1/4 cup cranberries, halved

mint leaves to garnish

Preheat oven to 375°. Place pumpkin seeds in a single layer in a 9-inch pie plate and bake until popped, about 10 to 15 minutes; stir seeds once or twice while cooking. When done cooking, coarsely grind pumpkin seeds in a grinder or blender.

Combine pumpkin seeds and millet in a clean bowl. Pour apple juice into a small pot, and bring to a boil; remove from heat, and pour over seed/millet mixture. Stir well to mix, and then pour into pie plate. Use a wooden spoon to push mixture up the sides of the pie plate.

In another bowl, combine grated apples, salt, cinnamon and arrowroot; mix well. Spoon this mixture over the millet crust; smooth with the back of a spoon. Top with halved cranberries, cover with foil and bake 45 minutes to 1 hour. Let cool completely before slicing.

DATES STUFFED WITH WALNUTS

8 pitted medjool or other large dates

8 walnut halves, split into thin slivers

With a knife, slit each date open enough to insert several slivers of walnut per date. Wrap in plastic wrap and chill.

Try this: Freeze stuffed dates and pack frozen into lunch boxes. They'll be thawed by lunch and delightfully cool.

CAROB MINT ICE CREAM

2 frozen bananas

½ to ⅓ cup water

2 Tbsp. nuts or 1 Tbsp. peanut butter

⅛ Tbsp. mint oil or peppermint flavoring

1/16 Tbsp. salt

1½ Tbsp. carob powder

Place all the ingredients in a blender or food processor, and whip until smooth. For a more solid ice cream, freeze for about 1 hour before serving.

"CHEESY" POPCORN

Air popped popcorn

Wheat free tamari

Nutritional yeast

Place tamari in a small pump spray bottle (you can find these in almost any pharmacy), and spray tamari on the popcorn. Sprinkle on the nutritional yeast, and enjoy.

Brunch Munch

Egg Alternatives & Grits Like You've Never Seen

"EGGS" FLORENTINE

Servings: 1

2 oz. firm tofu (½" thick cutlet)

1 tsp. each wheat free tamari,

Lemon juice, and filtered water

2 cups spinach leaves, packed fresh

(or about 10 oz. frozen)

¼ cup lemon sauce (see other recipe)

Fresh nutmeg and black pepper

⅛ cup wheat free tamari

Sauté the tofu in first liquids in a small skillet; sprinkle on spices. Cook both sides; set the tofu aside on another plate. Add spinach leaves and 1/8 cup tamari to the skillet; stir quickly over a medium high heat, only 3 to 4 minutes. Make a bed of spinach on each plate; place the tofu filet on top. Drizzle sauce on top.

BRUNCH SCRAMBLED "EGGS"

Servings: 2

1 Tbsp. tamari wheat free

2 Tbsp. filtered water or distilled water

1 garlic clove, pressed

½ onion, sliced

1 cup tofu

a dash of turmeric

1 drop toasted sesame oil

1 tomato, cut into wedges or seeded and chopped

Heat the tamari and filtered water in a wok or skillet; add the garlic; stir quickly. Add the onions and spices; sauté briefly until tender. Add the tofu; simmer 5 minutes. Toss in the tomato wedges 1 minute before serving.

SPICY TOMATO GRITS

½ cup chopped tomato

1 Tbsp. finely chopped fresh basil or 1 Tbsp. dried basil

¼ Tbsp. hot sauce or ¼ Tbsp. cayenne pepper

1 Tbsp. tomato paste

1 cup prepared grits

Prepare grits as instructed on the package; mix in other ingredients.

1 cup per serving.

PESTO GRITS

Add 3 heaping Tbsp. of any type of pesto sauce (see other recipe) to one cup grits.

ORIENTAL GRITS

2 tsp. grated fresh ginger or 1 tsp. dried ginger

1 Tbsp. fresh lemon juice

1 tsp. minced garlic or 2 tsp. chopped scallion

1 cup prepared grits

Prepare grits as instructed on the package; mix in other ingredients. One cup per serving.

MUSHROOM GRITS

2 Tbsp. olive oil

¼ cup any type mushroom

¼ cup chopped onion

Salt and pepper to taste

½ cup prepared grits

Sauté mushrooms and onion in oil until onions are golden brown. Prepare grits as instructed on the package. Mix ingredients together, and season to taste. One cup per serving.

CAJUN TOFU

Servings: 3 to 4

1 pound firm tofu

(Press between towels to rid tofu of water)

1 Tbsp. lemon juice

1 Tbsp. liquid aminos or wheat free/gluten free tamari

1½Tbsp. Cajun spice blend (see other recipe)

Slice the tofu into ½"thick filets, then cut each filet crosswise and lengthwise yielding 2" x 2" cutlets. Marinate the cutlets in the juice for a minimum of 30 minutes. Put the spice blend into a plastic bag, add tofu cutlets and gently shake the cutlets to coat them evenly.

Lay the tofu cutlets onto a broiling pan (ventilated so they will get crisp) on the top rack of the oven. Broil the top side for 7 to 9 minutes, turn and broil the bottom side for 7 to 9 minutes or barbecue.

CAJUN SPICE

1-3 tsp. cayenne pepper (mild, medium, hot)

1½tsp. black pepper, freshly ground

1½tsp. sea salt

2 tsp. (each) oregano, thyme, fennel, cumin, cardamom, garlic powder, chili powder and coriander

Whirl the spices in a blender, or mix all of the ingredients together by hand. Store in a glass jar, away from heat and light.

SCRAMBLED "EGGS" ANOTHER WAY

Servings: 2

½ cup onion, chopped

2 Tbsp. water

1 Tbsp. oil

2 cups firm tofu

2 Tbsp. chives, chopped

1 Tbsp. poultry seasoning

½ tsp. onion powder

1 tsp. nutritional yeast flakes

1 tsp. garlic powder

1 tsp. turmeric

½ tsp. lemon juice or salt

Sauté onion, water and oil in a pan. Add tofu, and mash with a fork until scrambled. (Take the water out of the tofu package, and discard it). Add chives, poultry seasoning, onion powder, yeast flakes, garlic powder, turmeric and lemon juice or salt. Heat until flavors are blended. Serve hot or cold as a sandwich filler.

A

B

C

D

H

I

J

N

O

T